Download the Gunner Goggles App Now!

Go to the App Store from your iPhone or iPad and search for **Gunner Goggles**

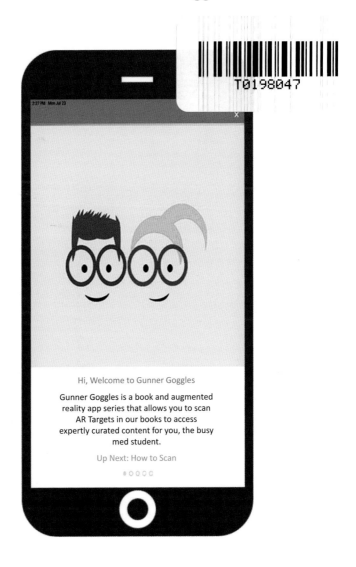

Each Gunner Goggles specialty has its own app; you can purchase other titles at:
ElsevierHealth.com/GunnerGoggles

GUNNER GOGGLES

Psychiatry

HONORS SHELF REVIEW

EDITORS:

Hao-Hua Wu, MD
Resident, Department of Orthopaedic Surgery
University of California–San Francisco
San Francisco, California

Leo Wang, MS, PhD
Perelman School of Medicine
University of Pennsylvania
Philadelphia, Pennsylvania

FACULTY EDITOR:

Olga Achildi, MD
Perelman School of Medicine
University of Pennsylvania
Philadelphia, Pennsylvania

ELSEVIER

ELSEVIER

1600 John F. Kennedy Blvd.
Ste 1800
Philadelphia, PA 19103-2899

GUNNER GOGGLES PSYCHIATRY, HONORS SHELF REVIEW   ISBN: 978-0-323-51039-4

Library of Congress Cataloging-in-Publication Data
Names: Wu, Hao-Hua, editor. | Wang, Leo, editor. | Achildi, Olga, editor.
Title: Gunner goggles psychiatry : honors shelf review / editors, Hao-Hua Wu,
    Leo Wang ; faculty editor, Olga Achildi.
Description: Philadelphia, PA : Elsevier, [2019] | Includes bibliographical references.
Identifiers: LCCN 2017046946 | ISBN 9780323510394 (pbk. : alk. paper)
Subjects: | MESH: Mental Disorders | Test Taking Skills | User-Computer Interface | Study Guide
Classification: LCC RC454 | NLM WM 18.2 | DDC 616.89--dc23 LC record available at https://lccn.loc.gov/2017046946

Executive Content Strategist: Jim Merritt
Content Development Manager: Lucia Gunzel
Publishing Services Manager: Patricia Tannian
Senior Project Manager: Cindy Thoms
Senior Book Designer: Maggie Reid

Printed in China

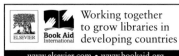

Working together to grow libraries in developing countries

www.elsevier.com • www.bookaid.org

Last digit is the print number: 9 8 7 6 5 4 3 2 1

Gunner Goggles Honors Shelf Review Series

Gunner Goggles Family Medicine	978-0-323-51034-9
Gunner Goggles Medicine	978-0-323-51035-6
Gunner Goggles Neurology	978-0-323-51036-3
Gunner Goggles Obstetrics and Gynecology	978-0-323-51037-0
Gunner Goggles Pediatrics	978-0-323-51038-7
Gunner Goggles Psychiatry	978-0-323-51039-4
Gunner Goggles Surgery	978-0-323-51040-0

Contributors

Anup Bhattacharya, MD
Resident Physician
Mallinckrodt Institute of Radiology
Washington University School of Medicine in St. Louis
St. Louis, Missouri
Substance-Related Disorders

James Janopaul-Naylor, BA
Perelman School of Medicine
University of Pennsylvania
Philadelphia, Pennsylvania
Schizophrenia and Other Psychotic Disorders

Thomas Knightly, MD
Resident Physician
Department of Psychiatry
Temple University School of Medicine
Philadelphia, Pennsylvania
Anxiety Disorders

Daniel Pustay, BA
Temple University School of Medicine
Philadelphia, Pennsylvania
Other Disorders/Conditions

Benjamin Yu, MD
Resident Physician
Department of Psychiatry
Yale School of Medicine
New Haven, Connecticut
Mood Disorders

Acknowledgments

"If I have seen further than others, it is by standing upon the shoulders of giants."
–Isaac Newton

We would like to thank the many exceptional innovators who helped transform our vision of *Gunner Goggles Psychiatry* into reality.

To our editorial team at Elsevier, thank you for your unrelenting support throughout the publication process. Jim Merritt believed in *Gunner Goggles* from day one and used his experience as an executive content strategist to point us in the right direction with respect to book proposal, product pitch and manuscript development. Margaret Nelson and Lucia Gunzel expertly guided us through manuscript submission and revision, no easy feat with two first-time authors. Maggie Reid collaborated with us closely to create the layout design and color schemes. Cindy Thoms and the copy editing team made sure our written content adhered to a high professional standard.

To the editors, authors, and student reviewers of *Gunner Goggles Psychiatry*, thank you for your scholarship and unwavering enthusiasm. Dr. Olga Achildi took time out of her busy clinical practice to meticulously edit each chapter, and she provided numerous invaluable insights on how we could improve quality and accuracy. A number of outstanding residents and medical students contributed to the content of this textbook and provided us feedback on high-yield topics for the NBME Psychiatry Subject Exam, notably Dr. Anup Bhattacharya, James Janopaul-Naylor, Dr. Thomas Knightly, Daniel Pustay, Dr. Benjamin Yu.

To our augmented reality (AR) team, thank you for your creativity and dedication during the development of the *Gunner Goggles* AR application. Nadir Bilici, Brian Mayo, Vlad Obsekov, Clare Teng, and Yinka Orafidiya helped us develop and test the initial *Gunner Goggles* AR prototype. Tammy Bui designed the *Gunner Goggles* logo and AR app icon.

We would also like to thank the Wharton Innovation Fund for awarding us seed money to help pursue development of *Gunner Goggles* AR.

You all continue to inspire us, and we are incredibly grateful and deeply appreciative for your support.

–Hao-Hua and Leo

Contents

Introduction

Hao-Hua Wu and Leo Wang

I. The Gunner's Guide to a Better Test Score

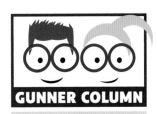

GUNNER COLUMN

Are you curious why certain classmates perform well on every exam? Are you frustrated by how few of these "gunner" peers share study secrets?

At *Gunner Goggles* (GG), our goal is to reveal and demystify. By integrating **augmented reality** (AR) into this review book, we **reveal** how some of the best students approach topics, conceptualize complex diseases, and efficiently allocate study time. By organizing each topic according to the National Board of Medical Examiners (NBME) format, we **demystify** exam content and the types of questions one can expect on test day.

Of the tests medical students strive to conquer, shelf exams boast the highest ratio of importance to the quality of study resources. For instance, performance on shelf exams typically informs final clerkship grades, which are the most important criteria on the medical school transcript for residency application. Yet, there is no single authoritative study resource for the shelf across all disciplines. Most importantly, no current book specifically targets shelf exam prep, so students must rely on miscellaneous resources and anecdotal advice to get the job done.

In light of this void in authoritative test prep, we have created the *Gunner Goggles* series to provide you with the most effective shelf exam testing resource. *GG* stands out for three important reasons.

First, readers have the opportunity to enhance understanding of important shelf topics by utilizing the AR features on each page. With an iPhone or iPad, users can download the *Gunner Goggles* AR iOS app and use it to turn book figures into three-dimensional (3D) images, access high-yield videos and view pertinent digital media. More on how AR technology works can be found on page 2.

Second, *Gunner Goggles* provides a plethora of tips on how to efficiently manage time when studying for the shelf. Mnemonics and strategies for how to approach difficult concepts can be found in the blue "Gunner

Column" to the right or left of each page. We also tell you how to **think** about these concepts so that medicine never feels like a laundry list of items you simply have to memorize.

Third, this review book is written and organized optimally for shelf exam test prep. Each chapter is organized according to the NBME Shelf Exam and United States Medical Licensing Examination (USMLE) Course Content outlines. In addition, a concise summary of how topics are tested prefaces each chapter.

As experts on the shelf exam, we understand how difficult it is to carve out time to study while juggling clinical responsibilities during your clerkship rotation. We also know that each student's learning curve is different based on the timing of the rotation (first block vs. last block), the year in medical school (MS3 vs. MD/PhD returning after graduate school), and future career interests (e.g., an aspiring orthopedic surgeon learning about obstetrics and gynecology). However, we believe that any student can perform well on the shelf with the right strategy and study resources.

We created this book anticipating the needs of all types of students, and hope that *Gunner Goggles* will be the most comprehensive, authoritative shelf exam review book that you ever use. We are confident that *Gunner Goggles* will enable you to achieve your test performance goals and stick it to your "gunner" classmates, whose advice, or lack thereof, you won't be needing after all.

II. Augmented Reality: A New Paradigm for Shelf Exam Test Prep

Think of AR as your best friend.

To use it, download the free *Gunner Goggles Psychiatry* application on your iPad or iPhone and create your own optional profile. Now with the *application* open, point your smart mobile camera at this page.

Notice how, on your camera, there are now links you can click on, 3D figures you can rotate, and a video you can watch. You have just unlocked the AR features for this page!

Take a moment to play around with these AR features on your smart mobile device. The way this works is that anytime you see the "Gunner Goggles" icon **gg** in the blue Gunner Column to the right or left, there is an AR feature accompanying the text with which you have the opportunity to interact with.

gg AR

Gunner Goggles Introduction Video

gg AR

Gunner Goggles Contact

Still not convinced? Here are three reasons why AR is your ideal study companion: presentation, evaluation, and community engagement.

Presentation

AR breaks the boundaries of how information can be presented in this textbook.

Traditionally, if you wanted to learn about a disease in a review book, you would be expected to read and memorize a block of text similar to the following:

"Huntington disease (HD) is a GABAergic neurodegenerative disorder that is caused by an autosomal dominant mutation leading to CAG repeats on chromosome 4. Patients typically present in the fourth and fifth decade of life with chorea, memory loss, caudate atrophy on neuroimaging, and motor impairment, depending on the variant. Although there is no cure for HD, the movement disorders associated with the disease, such as chorea, can be treated with drugs like tetrabenazine and reserpine to decrease dopamine release."

Having read (or most likely glazed) through that last paragraph, do you feel comfortable enough to answer questions about the genetics, presentation, and treatment of HD right now? A week from now? Three weeks from now when you have to take your shelf exam?

Here's where AR comes in. Use your *Gunner Goggles* app to check out how we're able to present HD in different, memorable ways.

For visual learners, here's a video of an effective HD mnemonic→

If you're an audio learner, here's a link to key points about HD for the shelf→

Forgot your neuroanatomy? Here's where the caudate is→

What's the difference between chorea, athetosis, and ballismus again? Chorea looks like this→

Now write a one-line description of HD in your own words in the margins of this page for future reference. It's much easier with AR, right? Like we said, your best friend.

gg AR
Huntington Disease Mnemonic

gg AR
Huntington Podcast

gg AR
The caudate nucleus is part of the basal ganglia

gg AR
Chorea patient example

Evaluation

The GG Psychiatry app has the potential to exponentially enhance how you can evaluate your own understanding of the material. Although not available with the first edition, we are in the process of developing a personalized question bank as well as a flashcards feature. Our vision is to allow you to scan a topic on the page for immediate access to relevant practice questions and flashcards. In future versions, you will also be able to create your own flashcard deck and track your mastery.

In addition the GG app can keep track of the AR Targets scanned and the Learning links viewed. These links are saved to a Link Library which you can view at any time. You can also like or dislike a Learning Link with an opportunity to provide us feedback for better resources available.

As development of the GG Psychiatry app is an ongoing process, we encourage and welcome your feedback. If you like the idea of having a personalized question bank and flashcard feature or have an idea for how we can improve the GG app to better serve your studying needs, please provide us feedback through an in-app message. You can also email us at GunnerGoggles@gmail.com.

Community Engagement

Studying for the shelf can be isolating. Our vision is to develop a feature in the GG Psychiatry that would allow you to connect with chapter authors and fellow readers. We are in the process of developing a medium in which shelf-related inquiries can be discussed among authors and readers through an optional short message system (SMS) feature.

Given that the community engagement feature is in development and unavailable for the first edition, we welcome your input on how we can connect you with the people who will enable your test day success.

To provide feedback, please scan the page and vote. You can also email us GunnerGoggles@gmail.com for any comments or suggestions.

Augmented Reality Frequently Asked Questions

"Since AR is integrated into *Gunner Goggles Psychiatry*, does this mean I have to pull out my iPad or iPhone for every page of the book?"

No, only if you need it. Some may use AR more than others, depending on their background and level of comfort with psychiatry. For instance, you may already have a solid understanding of HD and only need to read the text as a refresher. On the other hand, if you are less comfortable with HD, the AR features are there just in case.

gg AR

Gunner Goggles Forum

"Can't I just look up everything I don't know on my own? Why do I have to use the *Gunner Goggles* app?"

You can absolutely look things up on your own. But that takes time, and sometimes you can't find the best reference or mnemonic. We have already gone through the trouble of identifying potential sources of confusion for you and found the perfect resources. In the *Gunner Goggles* app, we have compiled the slickest and most concise resources one can use to better understand a topic. Videos, audio files, and images are first vetted by subject experts for accuracy of content. They are then evaluated by students like yourself for utility of content to enhance test performance. Only resources with the most Gunner votes are embedded into each page.

"What if a link doesn't work or I want something on the page to change?"

Please tell us! Another advantage of AR is that we can immediately receive and implement your feedback. Just use the *Gunner Goggles* app to text us your concerns and our tech support team will respond ASAP!

III. Study Smart: Mnemonics and Gunner Study Tips

Even with incredible AR features at your disposal, you won't be able to optimize exam performance unless you know how to study. Below are the four most important things one can do to study for the shelf under the time constraints imposed by clerkships.

Understand the Organizing Principle

The first most important piece of advice is to understand how a specific disease or concept fits into the big picture, which is the easiest way to both save time and perform well on the shelf. For instance, knowing the mechanism, diagnostic criteria, and treatment plan for HD will likely lead to only one correct answer on the test. However, understanding that HD exists on a spectrum of neurodegenerative disorders presenting with memory loss can enhance your ability to answer any question in which patient recall is an issue. Thus when you read about HD, be sure to differentiate it from dementia, Alzheimer disease, and amnesia, which are all disorders that can lead to memory impairment. Forcing yourself to make these connections and compare diseases among themselves is a relatively quick mental exercise that can greatly deepen your understanding of the material.

Create Effective Mnemonics

If you have a photographic memory, skip this section. For the rest of us mere mortals, the second most important piece of advice is the organizing principles (OP) of what constitutes a Gunner mnemonic, which are outlined below.

Mnemonics are important when

a. You have to learn a lot of material.
b. You want to teach something to your colleagues during morning rounds. Attendings and residents are always impressed when they can learn something from a medical student.
c. You want to remember something 15 years from now when you are working the 30th hour of a busy call day. OP for mnemonics are as follows:

1. Use the spelling of a name to your benefit (**Spell**)
Example:
   a. "Burkitt" lymphoma (Burkitt lymphoma), lep"thin" (leptin), "supraoptiuretic" nuclei (supraoptic nuclei that produces antidiuretic hormone)
   b. Tenofovir is the only NRTI nucleoTide
   c. We"C"ener's granulomatosis (GPA) for C-ANCA and Cyclophosphamide tx
2. Create an acronym that contains distinguishing syllables or letters of names (**Distinguish**)
Example:
   a. Chronic Alcoholics Steal PhenPhen and Nevar Rifuse Grisee Carbs (<u>Chronic alcohol</u> abuse + <u>St</u> John's wort + <u>phen</u>ytoin + <u>pheno</u>barb + <u>nevar</u>ipine + <u>rif</u>ampin + <u>grise</u>ofulvin + <u>carb</u>amazepine)
      • reinforce mnemonic by spelling the name of item-to-be-memorized accordingly
      • For example, "Refus"ampin, "Never"apine, "Greasy"ofulvin, "Carb"amazepine, etc.
      • This ties mnemonic OP 1 with mnemonic OP 2
3. Drawings help (**Draw**)
   Example: Trisomy 13 looks like polydactyly + cleft lip when the number 13 is rotated 90 degrees clockwise (the horizontal 1 is the extra digit, and the cleft of the horizontal 3 is the cleft lip)
4. Counting the letters of a word (**Count**)
   Example: Patau syndrome = 13 letters = Trisomy 13
5. Arrange acronym in alphabetical order (**Arrange**)
   Example: ABCDEF for diphtheria (ADP ribosylation, beta prophage, C Diphtheria, elongation factor 2)

Examples of instructors who practice this concept well are Dr. John Barone of Kaplan and Dr. Husain Sattar of Pathoma.

gg AR

Trisomy 13 mnemonic

On the flip side, here are examples of poor mnemonics (although you may remember them now given how they were highlighted in this text).

a. Blind as a bat, mad as a hatter, red as a beet, hot as Hades, dry as a bone, the bowel and bladder lose their tone, and the heart runs alone = poor mnemonic for anticholinergic syndrome
- This mnemonic forces you to memorize extra and extraneous things (like bat, beet, hare, and desert), which have nothing to do with anticholinergic syndrome.

b. WWHHHHIMP (withdrawal + wernicke + hypertensive crisis + hypoxia + hypoglycemia + hypoperfusion + intracranial bleed + meningitis/encephalopathy + poisoning) = poor mnemonic for causes of delirium
- Wait: how many H's does this mnemonic have again?

A good rule of thumb: if you can still remember a mnemonic under a high-pressure situation (attending pimps you) or after a 7-day period, then you have a winner.

Ultimately, the best mnemonics are the ones you invent and apply repeatedly. So use these mnemonic principles to give yourself a solid head start.

Devise a Study Schedule and Stick to It

The third most important piece of advice for the shelf is to create a study schedule at the beginning of the rotation and follow it. Rotations are draining, and often you may find yourself coming home after a 12-hour shift not wanting to study. However, if you are mentally committed to following a schedule, you will find creative ways to get studying done. For example, some students wake up an hour early to read before pre-rounds. Other students fit study material into their white coat and read during downtime.

Distinguish Rotation-Knowledge From Shelf-Knowledge

Most things you learn on rotation do not apply to the shelf exam and vice versa. For example, you may be able to impress your psychiatry attending by committing the National Institutes of Health (NIH) Stroke Scale to memory. However, with only 150 minutes to answer 100 lengthy questions on the shelf, diagnostic scores like that have no real utility.

Thus, you need to be able to compartmentalize, which is the fourth most important piece of advice. Knowing exactly what is needed for clinics and what is expected on the shelf can save you a lot of precious study time.

IV. Intro to the NBME Clinical Psychiatry Subject Exam

The Clinical Psychiatry NBME Shelf Exam is a 110-question computerized exam administered over a recommended course of 2 hours and 45 minutes, typically at the conclusion of one's psychiatry clerkship rotation. The test questions come from either retired Step 2 clinical knowledge (CK) questions or are written by a committee of faculty across the country. Thus, it is important to master shelf exam style questions to set yourself up nicely for Step 2 CK.

Unlike Step 1, shelf exam questions focus almost exclusively on disease processes rather than normal processes. That being said, the most high-yield normal process to know for the psychiatry shelf is normal aging, as question writers are known to present a question stem of normal aging phenomena and try to trick you with pathological answer choices.

According to the NBME, the exams are curved to a mean of 70 with a standard deviation of 8. The curve does not take into account the timing of rotation. For instance, students who take the exam during their first clerkship block will be held to the same statistical standard as students who take the exam during their fourth block. However, the NBME does release "quarterly norm information" to medical schools in order to make clerkship directors aware of the relationship between exam scores and rotation timing. Importantly, as of now, shelf exam scores are sent to the school directly; students cannot request their shelf exam score independent of their school. Although different psychiatry clerkships have different standards for determining grades, in general, each program has its own internally generated shelf exam cutoff score that one needs to achieve in order to be eligible for the highest clerkship grade (e.g., Honors). If this is the case, confirm the cutoff score with your clerkship director so that you have a reasonable performance goal to shoot for.

Students are expected to master content organized into the following categories:

General Principles, Including Normal Age-Related Findings and Care of the Well Patient	5%-10%
Behavioral Health	65%-70%
Nervous System & Special Senses	10%-15%

Other Systems, including Multisystem   5%-10%
 Processes & Disorders
Social Sciences   1%-5%

Behavioral Health is the largest section and is further broken down into several testable categories. These categories are not assigned percentages by the NBME but are as follows:

Behavioral Health - 65%-70%

- Normal processes, including adaptive behavioral responses to stress and illness
- Psychotic disorders
- Anxiety disorders
- Mood disorders
- Somatic symptoms and related disorders
- Factitious disorders
- Eating disorders and impulse control disorders
- Disorders originating in infancy/childhood
- Personality disorders
- Psychosocial disorders/behaviors
- Substance abuse disorders
- Adverse effects of drugs

Currently, the NBME Medicine Content Outline breaks down question types into three categories:

Physician Tasks (from 2016 Content Outline)

Diagnosis: Knowledge Pertaining to   65-70%
 History, Exam, Diagnostic Studies, &
 Patient Outcomes
Health Maintenance, Pharmacotherapy,   30%-35%
 Intervention, & Management

Diagnosis: Knowledge Pertaining to History, Exam, Diagnostic Studies, & Patient Outcomes - 65-70%
 Health Maintenance, Pharmacotherapy, Intervention, & Management - 30%-35%

However, devising a study plan from these three categories can be confusing. "Applying Foundational Science Concepts," for instance, is vague and difficult to prepare for. Instead, many students prefer to study according to Physician Tasks provided in older content outlines. Since every subject exam question asks about one of four things – 1) protocol for promoting health maintenance (Prophylaxis [**PPx**]), 2) the mechanism of disease (**MoD**), 3) steps to establishing a diagnosis (**Dx**), and 4) steps of disease management (**Tx/Mgmt**) – we recommend studying according to Physician Tasks from the 2016 Content Outline.

In addition, the NBME breaks down questions by Site of Care, including

- Ambulatory (65%-70%)
- Emergency Department (20%-30%)
- Inpatient (5%-10%)

Our recommendation is to not worry about site of care and focus on studying content related to Physician Tasks.

Gunner Goggles Psychiatry presents material to reflect how the NBME structures its shelf exams. Each chapter that follows falls into the main testable categories of General Principles (Chapter 2) or Mental Disorders (Chapters 3–10). Each disease is presented in a "PPx, MoD, Dx, and Tx/Mgmt" format, which represents the four physician tasks that the NBME can test you on. Since establishing a diagnosis is weighted especially heavily (55%–65%), the "Buzz Words" category shows readers how to quickly identify the disease process from just a few key words. The "Clinical Presentation" section services to more thoroughly describe the disease. However, it is important to note that Buzz Words are sufficient in correctly identifying the corresponding disease on the shelf. The detail provided in the Clinical Presentation section is only meant to augment your understanding, particularly if it is your first pass and you are unfamiliar with the material. However, by the end of studying, the focus should primarily be on Buzz Words.

Finally, here are six things to keep in mind when studying for the shelf.

1. If pressed for time, practice identifying disease processes only through "Buzz Words." For instance, a patient with anhedonia and sadness for over 2 weeks without the influence of substances should be considered to have major depressive disorder. Patients who are acutely combative and present to the emergency department (ED) with rotatory nystagmus have most likely taken PCP.

2. Many questions can double count for another exam topic. Watch out for cases that present like a psychiatric disease but are treated by other specialties (i.e., a patient presenting with pleasant, Lilliputian hallucinations secondary to Lewy Body dementia, which falls under the purview of neurology).

3. Make sure to begin doing questions early (e.g., 10 questions a day starting from day 1). Ideally you should make a second pass of the most high-yield questions.

4. For each question, write a one-line take-home point in an Excel spreadsheet. This makes for quick and easy review in the days leading up to the exam.
5. The questions will be a mix of the *Diagnostic and Statistical Manual of Mental Disorders* (DSM)-IV text revision (TR), and DSM V, since many of them were written before the newest iteration of the DSM was written. How do we know this? Asperger's, which is no longer a real diagnosis in DSM V, still appears from time to time on the psychiatry shelf. The most important thing is to focus on the core themes of a disease, or frankly what did not change with the new DSM. The most important principles are all covered in this text.
6. Lastly, remember the two salient OP of the psychiatry shelf as mentioned on page 5: (a) remember to rule out substance use with a urine drug screen; and (b) memorize the duration of symptoms for psychotic, mood, and anxiety-related disorders.

If any questions arise while studying, use the *Gunner Goggles* app to access the AR features embedded on each page.

Good luck and happy hunting.

—The *Gunner Goggles* Team

General Principles for the Psychiatry Shelf Exam

Hao-Hua Wu, Leo Wang, and Olga Achildi

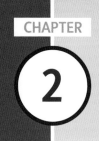

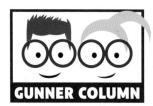

GUNNER COLUMN

Introduction

This chapter is high yield for two reasons. First, it contains many organizing principles that apply throughout the discipline of psychiatry, such as normal versus abnormal behavior. At the end of this chapter, you will be able to use clues, such as impairment of work and relationships, to discern which patients report normal behavior and only require reassurance. Second, this chapter highlights topics tested across different shelf exams. Questions pertaining to ethics can also appear on your medicine, family medicine, pediatrics, or neurology shelf. Questions about the mechanism, therapeutic use, or side effects of common psych drugs, such as haloperidol, will also appear on other exams. Thus learning this chapter well will not only help you answer 5–10 questions on your psychiatry shelf, but also help you with subsequent exams.

Students who have not had much exposure to psychiatric patients should expect to spend 8–12 hours taking multiple passes through this chapter. Those who are familiar with psychiatric patients, particularly the pharmacologic and psychotherapeutic treatments of disease as well as ethical principles, can expect to spend 4–8 hours on these subjects.

The General Principles chapter is organized into six sections: (1) Mental Status Examination (MSE), (2) Normal aging and behavior, (3) Abnormal aging and behavior, (4) Pharmacotherapies and psychotherapies, (5) Ethics, and (6) Gunner Practice. This chapter is intended for multiple passes so don't be discouraged if you feel overwhelmed after the initial read.

How to Examine a Psychiatric Patient: The Mental Status Exam

If you already know the MSE through your didactics or clinical experience, feel free to skip this section. However, if you are previewing for your rotation, become familiar with the general format of the MSE as well as the adjectives and nouns one can use to describe a patient evaluated for psychiatric disease. This subsection should take no longer than 30 minutes to review.

To be clear, you will not be asked specifically about the MSE nor be asked to describe the mental status of a patient on the shelf. However, the shelf may frequently include the results of the patient's MSE as important clues (e.g., flat affect, flight of ideas) to the diagnosis.

Mental Status Exam

The MSE contains 11 essential components: (1) appearance, (2) attitude, (3) behavior, (4) speech, (5) mood, (6) affect, (7) thought process, (8) thought content, (9) cognition, (10) insight, and (11) judgment. While many institutions have different variations of the MSE, the one presented here will give you a strong foundation of how health providers describe a psychiatric patient.

Appearance: As it sounds, this is used to describe your first impression of the patient. Information can include age, sex, type of dress, kempt versus unkempt, cleanliness, nutritional status, etc. Depressed patients may present as unkempt. Manic patients may dress or present themselves in bright colors (e.g., bright-colored shirt/pants/jacket, bright lipstick, brightly dyed hair).

Attitude: This describes the patient's attitude towards responding to questions: cooperative versus uncooperative; friendly versus unfriendly; and pleasant versus unpleasant versus hostile. Actively psychotic patients are often uncooperative. Patients with borderline personality disorder can be hostile to some and friendly to others (e.g., splitting).

Behavior: This is how the patient physically behaves, with a focus on motor. This is the same as how one would describe the "general" appearance of a patient for a physical exam. It includes details like eye contact, motor (e.g., any abnormal tics, twitches, dystonia, akathisia, tar dyskinesia, movement disorders). Psychotic patients often have poor eye contact. Patients on antipsychotic medication (e.g., haloperidol) may exhibit tardive dyskinesia.

Speech: This requires a description of the patient's speech in four categories:
1. Quantity: overly talkative, poverty of speech
2. Rate: pressured, rapid, slow
3. Volume: soft, loud, monotone
4. Rhythm: regular, irregular, appropriate inflections, pauses

Affect and mood video

Poverty of speech is one of the negative symptoms of schizophrenia. Pressured speech is a Buzz Word for a patient enduring a manic/hypomanic episode.

Mood: Subjective emotion. Unlike speech or behavior, one's mood is a patient-reported subjective emotion elicited through a question. Your attending may ask you to present a patient's mood as his or her response to the question "How is your mood right now?" or "How are you feeling today?" For example, a depressed patient may state "I am sad today."

Affect: This is the patient's objective emotion and includes the observation of their reaction to external stimuli, such as conversation. This can be described with respect to
1. appropriateness to situation (appropriate vs. non-appropriate)
2. range of emotion (broad or restricted)
3. intensity (blunted, flat expression)
4. quality (e.g., indifferent, hostile, anxious, animated, dysphoric, euphoric, spontaneous)
5. fluctuation: continuous, labile

Schizophrenic patients often have flat affects. Patients in the middle of a major depressive episode may appear dysphoric.

Thought Process: This is a description of the **flow** of patient narrative. When patients answer their questions, are their stories linear? Circumferential? Tangential? Flight ideas? Do sentences fail to connect to one another (loose association)?

Examples of thought processes used to describe patients:
1. Circumstantial: the patient circles around the point, makes the point, but includes many unnecessary details
2. Tangential: the patient talks about a different topic altogether
3. Derailment: the patient stays on a topic but then is no longer on that topic
4. Loose association: the patient goes from one point to another but there are NO associations between the two points
5. Flight of ideas: the patient jumps really fast from topic to topic, but they are somehow related
6. Clanged association: patient's thoughts that are connected based on how words sound, clang tang, psych, trick; can be a symptom of psychosis
7. Echolalia: repeating sounds, jingles
8. Neologism: making up new words

Thought Content: The patient focuses specifically on thought content. This is the category to elicit suicidal ideation and homicidal ideation. Also, can record delusions and hallucinations.

Cognition: Attention (e.g., awake, alert, and oriented to patient, place, and time) and memory. This is used to rule out (r/o) neurological disease, such as dementia.

Insight: The patient's ability to articulate their condition and reason for admission. Can they state why they are in the hospital? Do they know why? Are they compliant with treatment?

- Impaired insight in schizophrenics and dementia

Judgment: This describes the appropriateness of judgment. Can a patient respond to a normal scenario (e.g., What would you do if you found five bucks on the ground?).

Example of How MSE May Be Presented During Rounds:

History of present illness: Mr. D is a 25-year-old Caucasian male with a history of opiate dependence, alcohol abuse, benzodiazepine abuse, marijuana abuse, depression, and anxiety who presents to the emergency room 2 days after putting a stop to a 3-week-long opiate binge.

MSE:

Appearance: Appropriately groomed, alert, appears stated age

Attitude: Cooperative, pleasant, friendly

Behavior: Sitting comfortably in a chair, making appropriate eye contact

Speech: Regular in rate, rhythm, quantity, spontaneity, and latency

Mood: "Above average"

Affect: Euthymic, expansive, congruent to stated mood

Thought Process: Sometimes circumstantial, but largely linear, logical, goal-directed

Thought Content: Is concerned about setting a good example for his younger brothers, endorses SI in the past but currently denies SI, HI, AVH, and paranoid delusions

Cognition: A&Ox3, 3/3 memory, able to spell LEARN backwards

Insight: Good, able to clearly articulate his condition and what brought him to the hospital

Judgment: Good, recognized that stealing from best friend was inappropriate, and made appropriate changes

---

QUICK TIPS

auditory hallucinations →
psychosis
  visual hallucinations →
delirium
  tactile hallucinations→
withdrawal of substances

FOR THE WARDS

SI = suicidal ideation; HI = homicidal ideation; AVH = auditory and visual hallucinations

Adaptive Behavior Response to Stress and Illness

Understanding normal will help you understand abnormal.

While the shelf exams focus primarily on testing disease processes, normal aging, behavior, and adaptive responses to stress and illness fall under the "General Principles" category that comprises 5%–10% of the Psychiatry shelf. This topic can also appear on the Neurology, Medicine, and Family Medicine shelf exams. By the end of this chapter, you need to be able to delineate normal aging as well as the four mature responses to stress.

Normal Aging

Buzz Words: Decreased Achilles tendon reflex (aka "1+" or less) + difficulty remembering if not enough rest + awakens early in the morning + increasing stiffness + presbyopia + presbycusis → normal aging

Clinical Presentation: The key to answering questions about normal aging is being able to understand what signs and symptoms are age appropriate. The classic example is a more than 65-year-old patient coming in for a regular health maintenance exam who is sleeping less, found to have 1+ Achilles reflex, but no real chief complaint. Normal aging:

- Does not predispose one in it of itself to bruising
- Increases predisposition to autoimmunity due to exposure of more antigens that increase chance for the development of antigens that may recognize self
- Diminishes cough reflex → predisposes one to aspiration pneumonia
- Decreases rapid eye movement (REM) latency, meaning they go into REM sleep quicker, but total time spent in REM is reduced. Time spent in stage 1 and 2 increases, but deeper sleep decreases, thus reducing sleep efficiency
- Decreases with sleep time
- Decreases testosterone, bone density, and glomerular filtration rate (GFR)
- Does not affect thyroid function

PPx: N/A

MoD: N/A

Dx: N/A

Tx/Mgmt: N/A

Poor sleep hygiene practices include:
1. Drinking more caffeine
2. Smoking
3. Exercising **late in the day**
4. Eating a late dinner
5. Working late on laptop

Response to Stress and Illness: Mature Defense Mechanisms

Patients respond to stress and illness in many different ways: 4 are mature; 15 are immature. Patients who employ altruism, humor, sublimation, and suppression channel negative emotions into a productive outlet (mature defenses). Immature defense mechanisms, on the other hand, diminishes one's chance of success and will be covered in the "Maladaptive Behavior" subsection below.

Mature Defense Mechanisms

1. **Suppression**: The patient puts unwanted feelings aside to cope with reality. This has a very high yield on the shelf because it is frequently compared to repression, which is an immature defense mechanism that blocks upsetting feelings from entering consciousness. The easiest way to differentiate between the two is to determine whether or not the patient consciously decided not to think about a negative experience. Patients who are conscious about their decision not think about a stressor employ suppression, which allows them to deal with the negative emotions after the task at hand is complete. Patients who do not consciously make the decision not to think about a stressor but have "forgotten" about the stressor entirely are repressing their emotions, which leads to present maladaptive behavior (e.g., forgetting a close relative's funeral) and potential future emotional outbursts.

2. **Sublimation**: The patient channels impulses into socially acceptable behaviors. This is the second most commonly tested mature defense mechanism because the behavior described is not obvious from the name. An example includes a patient who redirects anger into playing a violent sport, such as rugby or wrestling.

3. **Altruism**: The patient avoids negative feelings by helping others. There is no financial incentive for these acts of kindness.
4. **Humor**: The patient uses humor to avoid uncomfortable feelings. Humor diffuses tension and helps redirect energy towards a common goal.

Maladaptive Behavior Response to Stress and Illness

So, what is maladaptive behavior? On the shelf, it means behavior that disrupts one's ability to participate in activities of daily living and gainful employment. For instance, people who employ one of the 15 immature defense mechanisms to cope with stress are less likely to be productive in their personal and professional life. However, it is important to recognize that normal people (i.e., folks who do not meet the threshold for disease) cope with immature defense mechanisms all the time. You may also recognize many in yourself (i.e., intellectualization when dealing with the death of a loved one), and that is OK. Using immature defense mechanisms doesn't mean there is something wrong with you.

However, many disorders manifest in very characteristic ways. Splitting, for instance, is classically associated with borderline personality disorder. Acting out is frequently seen in individuals with conduct and antisocial personality disorder.

In addition, several pathologic processes are associated with maladaptive behavior to stress and illness. In this subsection, we will cover the ones most commonly seen on the shelf: kleptomania and hoarding disorder.

Immature Defense Mechanisms

1. **Splitting**: Patients who see others as all bad or all good and act accordingly. This is the most high yield immature defense mechanism because it is pathognomonic for borderline personality disorder. This presents as a patient who is very nice to one care provider while being very mean to another. This is indisputably the most commonly tested immature defense mechanism on the shelf exam.
2. **Somatization**: Patients who transform emotional conflicts into physical symptoms. This is also high yield, since this is a behavior frequently seen in patients with somatization disorders.

3. **Dissociation**: Patients who disrupt memory, identity, and consciousness to cope with an event. This is good to know for the shelf because there is a set of disorders in which patients exhibit symptoms of dissociation.

4. **Displacement**: Patients who transfer feelings to a more acceptable object. Frequently tested. The classic example is a resident who is mad at the attending, but takes out that anger on a medical student.

5. **Repression**: Patient blocks upsetting feelings from entering consciousness. As mentioned above, repression is frequently compared to suppression, so will frequently be tested. Also, it is sometimes compared to denial, which is an immature defense in which the patient completely denies an aspect of reality.

6. **Denial**: Patient behaves as if an aspect of reality does not exist. Frequently compared to suppression and repression. This is only an immature defense where the event that's prompting negative feelings is completely denied. Even patients who repress or suppress feelings will admit that the event had occurred.

7. **Acting out**: Patient avoids unacceptable feelings by behaving badly. This is seen in antisocial and conduct disorder.

8. **Regression**: Patient reverts to earlier developmental stage. This is different from patients with developmental delay, who never reach an appropriate developmental stage in the first place.

9. **Reaction formation**: Patient responds in a manner opposite to one's actual feelings. This is a frequently tested defense mechanism because the meaning is not obvious in the name.

10. **Rationalization**: Patient justifies behavior to avoid challenging reality. One of the most common coping mechanisms you will encounter on the wards.

11. **Projection**: Patient projects one's own feelings towards another. A classic example is the angry patient who erroneously thinks everyone else around him is angry.

12. **Isolation of affect**: Patient separates thought from emotion. On MSE, the patient's affect would be stated as "incongruent" to the patient's mood.

13. **Intellectualization**: Patient uses intellect to avoid confronting uncomfortable emotions. This is frequently employed by physicians.

99 AR

Defense mechanisms explained by stick figures

14. **Fantasy**: Patient substitutes imaginary scenarios for troubling ones. Be sure to rule out delusional disorder.
15. **Distortion**: Patient alters perception of upsetting reality so that it is more acceptable.

A. Kleptomania

Buzz Words:
- Steals objects + stolen object not used or needed + low monetary value of stolen goods + leads to dysfunction in work and play → Kleptomania
- Repetitive failure to resist stealing impulse + feels guilt or remorse + anxiety before theft; relief of anxiety after theft → Kleptomania

Clinical Presentation: Kleptomania is a disorder defined by the uncontrollable urge to steal objects of little monetary value. This is considered a disorder stemming from maladaptive behavior since stealing is prompted by anxiety and perpetuated by poor coping mechanisms. The patient can be of any age or gender, but is typically seen exclusively in the outpatient setting. The most high-yield fact is that cognitive behavioral therapy (CBT) is used to treat kleptomania.

PPx: N/A
MoD: N/A
Dx: (1) MSE
Tx/Mgmt: (2) CBT

B. Hoarding Disorder

Buzz Words: Does not discard possessions regardless of worth + cluttered spaces that disrupts daily life at home + anxiety related to discarding possession + feels distress

Clinical Presentation: Patients with hoarding disorder hoard items and cannot bring themselves to discard items at the cost of daily living. This is not associated with age or gender, but is hereditary and exacerbated by stress. Make sure to r/o other disorders through thorough MSE.

PPx: N/A
MoD: N/A
Dx: (1) MSE
Tx/Mgmt: (1) CBT and selective serotonin reuptake inhibitor (SSRI)

Pharmacotherapy and Psychotherapy

Pharmacologic and psychotherapeutic treatment of psychiatric disease is the most high-yield subsection of this chapter. Remember to refer to these organizing principles

---

QUICK TIPS

Shoplifting unneeded items + guilt → Kleptomania

Theft for personal gain + patient capable of feeling guilt → Shoplifting

Theft for personal gain + patient not capable of feeling guilt → Antisocial Personality Disorder

Expensive item stolen + pressured speech + lack of sleep + grandiosity → manic episode (impulsivity)

MNEMONIC

A lot of letters in SSRI; SSRI seen as "hoarding" letters

again and again through your course of clerkship training. This material is meant to be digested after several passes so don't be discouraged if you cannot master it on your first pass.

To be successful, be sure to know the four neurotransmitters targeted in psychotherapy:

1. acetylcholine: nucleus basalis of Meynert; dementia
2. dopamine: high dopamine levels suspected in psychotic patients; low levels suspected in attention deficit hyperactivity disorder (ADHD) and Parkinson's
3. norepinephrine: seen in locus coeruleus and implicated in anxiety and mood
4. serotonin: seen in raphe nuclei; decreased in depression

This subsection presents (1) antipsychotics, (2) antidepressants, (3) mood stabilizers, (4) anxiolytics (benzos), and (5) psychotherapy treatments.

Antipsychotics

Antipsychotics can be divided into typical (first generation) and atypical (second generation) drugs. Commonly tested typical antipsychotics include haloperidol and chlorpromazine (first antipsychotic made); atypicals include olanzapine, clozapine, risperidone, quetiapine, ziprasidone, and aripiprazole.

The majority of antipsychotics block the D2 receptor in the central nervous system (CNS). It is thought an abnormal increase in dopamine in the mesolimbic pathway exacerbates positive symptoms of schizophrenia. On the shelf, antipsychotics, like haloperidol, are frequently used to treat delirium, a fact that can also be appreciated in the Neurology and Medicine shelf.

For antipsychotics, the number four is your friend. Four is the number of pathways where D2 receptors are located:

1. Mesocortical: too little dopamine = negative symptoms, for example, poor hygiene, flat affect
2. Mesolimbic: too much dopamine = positive symptoms, for example, AVH, delusions
3. Nigrostriatal: too little dopamine = extrapyramidal symptoms (EPS), for example, acute dystonic reaction, akathisia, and drug-induced Parkinsonism, tardive dyskinesia
4. Tubuloinfundibular: too little dopamine = prolactin-induced symptoms, for example, galactorrhea, gynecomastia. This is because dopamine inhibits prolactin release.

FOR THE WARDS

Neuroleptics = antipsychotic medication

9g AR

Video of EPS in patients

Four also describes the timing of EPS symptoms, which are frequently tested side effects of antipsychotics:
- Acute dystonia = 4 hours
- Akathisia = 4 days
- Parkinsonian signs (e.g., bradykinesia) = 4 weeks
- Tardive dyskinesia = 4 months

In addition to EPS, neuroleptic malignant syndrome (NMS) is the second most commonly tested antipsychotic side effect. Unlike EPS, NMS can occur at any time during the course of treatment. It presents classically in patients who take antipsychotics (e.g., prochlorperazine, droperidol) or metoclopramide and present with Fever, Altered mental status, Leukocytosis, Tremor, Elevated creatine phosphokinase (CPK) and Rigidity. The mnemonic is FALTER. This is an emergent side effect, which is why it is so frequently tested. NMS is treated by (1) discontinuing the offending drug, (2) supportive treatment with a cooling blanket, and (3) dopamine agonists (e.g., ropinirole, dantrolene, bromocriptine).

Be sure to know how to differentiate NMS from malignant hypertension and thyrotoxicosis. Malignant hypertension, for instance, is a deadly side effect of succinyl choline in genetically predisposed patients leading to muscle rigidity, arrhythmia, fever, metabolic acidosis, and respiratory acidosis. Thyrotoxicosis, on the other hand, can present with high fever, vomiting, and diarrhea in a patient with suspected thyroid pathology in the setting of a recent fever or biological insult.

The third most important group of antipsychotic side effects to remember are the anti-HAM: anti-Histamine, anti-Alpha1, anti-Muscarinic. Different antipsychotics lead to different anti-HAM responses. The general rule is that typical > atypical in the severity of anti-HAM effects. Within typical antipsychotics, low-potency (e.g., chlorpromazine) leads to more anti-HAM effects than medium- and high-potency.

The final general side effect of antipsychotics worth memorizing is that they lower seizure threshold and prolong QTc, particularly the atypical ziprasidone.

Typical antipsychotics antagonize D2 receptors only, and are sorted by three categories of potency:
1. High-potency typicals have **high** D2 action, **low** anti-HAM action, but **high** EPS incidence. Haloperidol can be used to treat Huntington's and Tourette's. Can also be used for pregnant women who are psychotic.
   Examples: haloperidol, pimozide (prolonged QT), loxapine, trifluoperazine, thiothixene

2. Medium-potency have a mix of anti-HAM and EPS side effects and are rarely tested. Examples include perphenazine.

3. Low-potency typicals have **low** D2 action, **high** anti-HAM, but **low EPS** incidence. Examples include chlorpromazine and thioridazine. This is frequently tested because of other side effects outside of anti-HAM, EPS, NMS, and seizure threshold. Chlorpromazine can cause obstructive jaundice and a purple, gray, metallic rash over sun-exposed areas. Thioridazine can cause pigmentary retinopathy and prolonged QTc.

Atypical antipsychotics antagonize both D2 and 5HT2a. They were created to mitigate negative symptoms and to quickly dissociation off of D2 receptors to allow for normal physiology after therapeutic effect. Atypicals are less likely to cause anti-HAM side effects, but are more likely to cause metabolic syndrome. Examples of atypicals include olanzapine, clozapine, risperidone, quetiapine, ziprasidone, and aripiprazole. Unlike typicals, atypicals are not grouped by category and must be considered individually:

Olanzapine → highest risk of metabolic syndrome

Risperidone → atypical with highest risk for EPS and prolactin-induced side effects

Clozapine → agranulocytosis, seizures, hypotension, cardiomyopathy, and sialorrhea; used as a drug of last resort; tested on many shelf exams because of risk of agranulocytosis; monitor with complete blood count (CBC) every week for 6 months; if patient has **sialorrhea**, treat with clonidine; be careful of adding more alpha blockers because clozapine already has alpha activity and will exacerbate orthostasis

Quetiapine → orthostasis, sedation, cataracts; very often used for sleep; slit lamp exam q6 months to screen for cataracts; safest one to use for Lewy body dementia due to high dissociation constant

Paliperidone → extended release, risperidone metabolite; so has risperidone side effects

Ziprasidone → weight neutral, prolongs QTc

Aripiprazole → weight neutral, akathisia; partial DA agonist, 5HT1a partial agonist, and 5HT2a antagonist; no risk of metabolic syndrome; patients may **decompensate** because medication can upregulate dopamine due to agonist activity

Antidepressants

The treatment of depression is based on the monoamine theory, which states that depleted levels of serotonin,

---

QUICK TIPS

Chlorpromazine = purple, grey, metallic rash over sun-exposed areas + jaundice. Famously taken by Mike Tyson. Can remember by picturing Mike Tyson with bruise-like rash and eyes that suggest jaundice.

QUICK TIPS

5-HT = 5-hydroxytrptamine receptors that bind serotonin

AR

Fast-off-D2 theory of atypicals

FOR THE WARDS

Clozapine is the only antipsychotic drug shown to decrease suicide risk. Lithium is another.

QUICK TIPS

The only two therapies used to decrease suicide in schizophrenics are clozapine and electroconvulsive therapy.

QUICK TIPS

Risk of metabolic syndrome: olanzapine > clozapine > risperidone > quetiapine

MNEMONIC

Olanzapine starts with O, the shape you become when you take it

dopamine, and norepinephrine in the CNS are responsible for depression. Antidepressants were created to modify these three neurotransmitters: serotonin, norepinephrine, and dopamine. For example, there are some drugs that affect the synapse concentration of 5HT alone (e.g., SSRI, buspirone), 5-HT and NE (serotonin-norepinephrine reuptake inhibitor [SNRI], tricyclic antidepressant (TCA), monoamine oxidase inhibitors [MAOI]), NE and dopamine (e.g., modafinil), and NE alone (e.g., mirtazapine). The purpose of this subsection is to provide you with an appreciation of the variation in antidepressant therapy, including electroconvulsive therapy (ECT).

A. SSRIs

Examples: Fluoxetine, sertraline, citalopram, escitalopram, fluvoxamine, and vilazodone

> You do not have to memorize the names of these drugs nor their brand names. Just be mindful of the following examples when specific SSRIs were tested:
> - Fluoxetine is the only one indicated in children and is safe during pregnancy
> - Fluvoxamine is first-line treatment for obsessive-compulsive disorder (OCD) and has a risk of fulminant hepatic failure

Indications: Depression, anxiety

Buzz Words: Hyperthermia + Autonomic instability + Rigidity + Myoclonus + Encephalopathy + Diaphoresis → SSRI intoxication (serotonin syndrome).

> Flu-like symptoms, Insomnia, Nausea, Imbalance, Sensory Disturbance, Hyperarousal→ SSRI withdrawal

Mechanism: Inhibits serotonin reuptake, thereby increasing serotonin concentration in the synapse; acts on the following receptors

> 5HT-1a → possible locus of depressive symptoms
> 5HT-2a, 5HT2c → initially presents with headaches, jitteriness; long term, presents with decreased libido, insomnia
> 5HT3, 5HT4 → gastrointestinal (GI) symptoms, such as N/V and diarrhea

Side Effects:
1. Common side effects pertain to sex and food.
   - Patients often report sexual dysfunction; treat by adding or switching to bupropion
   - Patients also report GI upset
2. The side effects can be understood through the 5-HT receptors targeted by SSRIs.

3. Patients who take too much SSRI or mix SSRI with MAO-inhibitors are HARMED: **H**yperthermia, **A**utonomic instability, **R**igidity, **M**yoclonus, **E**ncephalopathy, **D**iaphoresis
4. Patients who discontinue SSRIs present with FINISH: **F**lu-like symptoms, **I**nsomnia, **N**ausea, **I**mbalance, **S**ensory Disturbance, **H**yperarousal

B. MAOIs

Examples: Nonselective = isocarboxazid, phenelzine, hydracarbazine, tranylcypromine; selective MAO-A = moclobemide; MAO-B = rasagiline, selegiline
- isoniazid also has weak MAO-I properties

Indications: Depressed patient refractory to SSRI and TCAs → treat with MAOIs
Atypical depression → treat with MAOIs
Buzz Words:
- Patient prescribed MAOI + consumed liver or cheese (tyramine-rich) + muscle rigidity + arrhythmia + fever + metabolic acidosis + respiratory acidosis → malignant hypertension
- Patient prescribed MAOI + recent SSRI or TCA use + hyperthermia + autonomic instability + rigidity + myoclonus + encephalopathy + diaphoresis → serotonin syndrome

Mechanism: upregulates all monoamines (S, NE, D) by **irreversibly** binding to MAO-A and/or B. MAO-A metabolizes S, NE, and D. MAO-B metabolizes D.
Side Effects:
1. Hypertensive crises 2/2 excess NE
   - avoid tyramine because tyramine is a precursor to norepinephrine!
   - tyramine including foods (include cheese and liver)
   - also can be caused by ephedrine or meperidine, buspirone, levodopa
   - treat with **phentolamine** (alpha antagonist) or chlorpromazine for hypertensive emergencies
   - **clonidine** can be used for PPx to lower blood pressure when headache starts
2. Serotonin syndrome (e.g., if concomitant TCA or SSRI use)
3. Adrenergic side effects, such as orthostasis and cardiac arrhythmia
4. Hypertension if paired with sympathomimetics or buspirone
5. Preeclampsia in pregnancy
6. NMS when paired with SSRIs

99 AR
Overview of drug treatment for depression

FOR THE WARDS
Methylene blue is a reversible MAOI but is not used as an antidepressant

FOR THE WARDS
2-week washout needed after last dose of MAOI before prescribing SSRI or TCA

C. Tricyclic Antidepressants

Examples: Amitriptyline, imipramine, nortriptyline (secondary amine metabolite), desipramine (secondary amine metabolite)

Indications: Depression
- imipramine treats enuresis
- nortriptyline treats elderly depression
- clomipramine treats OCD
- amitriptyline and desipramine treats pain syndrome

Buzz Words: High blood pressure (hypertensive crisis)

Mechanism: (1) Sodium channel blocker, (2) L-type calcium channel blocker, (3) blocks S, NE reuptake transporters, thereby increasing NE and S in synapse

Side Effects:
1. 3 C's of TCA: Convulsions, Coma and Cardiac arrhythmia
2. Anti-HAM
3. Cardiotoxicity
4. Prolonged QRS >100 ms on ECG → arrhythmia → torsades de pointes
5. VFib = most common cause of death
   a. to prevent torsades, give activated charcoal if 1–2 hours; give sodium bicarb if greater than 2 hours
6. Amoxapine with worse antipsychotic side effects because metabolite of loxapine and tetracyclic TCA
   - secondary amines are less anticholinergic and can be given to elderly (desipramine, protriptyline, nortriptyline)
   - tertiary amines = worst anticholinergic properties

D. SNRIs

Examples: Venlafaxine, duloxetine, vortioxetine, levomilnacipran

Indications: Comorbid pain syndrome, neuropathic pain, diabetic neuropathy
- venlafaxine can be used for GAD, social anxiety

Buzz Words: High blood pressure + St. John's wort + generalized anxiety disorder (GAD) treated with venlafaxine → discontinue (d/c) St. John's wort

Mechanism: Inhibits reuptake of serotonin and norepinephrine to increase their concentration in the synapse
- dose increased by concomitant St. John's wort use

Side Effects: (1) NE side effects (orthostasis, cardiac arrhythmias), (2) serotonin side effects (N/V, diarrhea, loss of libido), and (3) withdrawal symptoms similar to SSRI withdrawal

---

gg AR

Effect of TCA on ECG

FOR THE WARDS

Not needed for the shelf, but during your rotation, be aware that venlafaxine effects vary by dose: <150 pro-serotonergic; 150–300 adds NE action, >300 mg elevates dopamine.

E. Serotonin Antagonist and Reuptake Inhibitors (SARI)

Examples: Trazodone, nefazodone
- do not confuse trazodone with tramadol (which is a weak mu-opioid receptor agonist)

Indications: (1) Sleep
- use nefazodone for decreased sexual dysfunction

Buzz Words: Priapism + PMHx of difficulty with sleep + treatment with trazodone → d/c trazodone

Mechanism:
1. antagonist of 5HT2 receptor so downregulates 5HT2 activity
2. **reuptake** antagonist of 5HT1a so upregulates 5HT1A activity
3. Partial 5HT1a agonist

Side Effects:
1. Priapism (trazodone)
2. Fatal hepatitis (nefazodone)

> **MNEMONIC**
> Trazodone = Trazo**bone** because of the risk of priapism

> **QUICK TIPS**
> 5HT-1a → possible locus of depressive symptoms
> 5HT-2a, 5HT2c → initially presents with headaches, jitteriness; long term, presents with decreased libido, insomnia
> 5HT3, 5HT4 → GI symptoms, such as N/V and diarrhea

F. Alpha-2 Antagonists

Examples: Mirtazapine

Indications: (1) Depression, (2) insomnia, (3) cachectic, (4) GAD, and (5) posttraumatic stress disorder (PTSD)

Buzz Words: N/A

Mechanism: (1) Antagonizes alpha 2 receptor which in turn upregulates NE and 5HT; (2) anti-HAM at low doses

Side Effects: (1) Increased appetite, (2) increased sleep

> **99 AR**
> Studies show that certain alpha2 receptors are norepinephrine release inhibitors, so if an alpha2 receptor is activated, no NE release; but if alpha2 is inhibited, NE is released because disinhibited.

G. Serotonin Partial Agonist

Examples: Buspirone (do not confuse with bupropion, which is a norepinephrine/dopamine reuptake inhibitors [NDRI])

Indications: (1) GAD

Buzz Words: Two drugs proven to decrease suicide risk → buspirone and clozapine

Mechanism: (1) Partially agonizes 5HT1a receptor

Side Effects: (1) Sedation, (2) dizziness, (3) GI disturbance

H. NDRI

Examples: Bupropion, modafinil

Indications: (1) Quit smoking/decrease craving (bupropion), (2) narcolepsy (modafinil), (3) depression (especially if the patient wants to avoid sexual dysfunction), and (4) social anxiety disorder

Buzz Words: Male patient cannot maintain erection + depression + long-term treatment with SSRI → switch to SSRI to bupropion

Mechanism: (1) Inhibit reuptake of NE and dopamine so upregulates NE and dopamine in the synapse

Side Effects: (1) Lowers seizure threshold, (2) worsens psychosis by upregulating dopamine, and (3) anxious and jittery

I. Norepinephrine Reuptake Inhibitor

Examples: Reboxetine, atomoxetine

Indications: (1) ADHD

Buzz Words: Treatment for ADHD refractory to methylphenidate → reboxetine or atomoxetine

Mechanism: (1) Inhibits reuptake of NE so upregulates NE in the synapse

Side Effects: (1) Tremor, and (2) tachycardia (NE side effects)

J. Electroconvulsive Therapy

ECT is a procedure and not by any means part of the class of antidepressant drugs. However, it is included here because it is an important therapeutic agent for depression that is frequently tested. 80% remission for MDD.

Indications: (1) Refractory depression, (2) MDD with psychosis, and (3) treatment-resistant psychosis or mania

Buzz Words: Patient with depression refractory to pharmacotherapy → try ECT

Depression refractory to pharmacotherapy + space-occupying lesion → avoid ECT

Mechanism: (1) Unknown how it modulates depressive symptoms

Side Effects: (1) Memory loss (transient)

Mood Stabilizer

The mechanism of mood stabilizers with respect to psychiatric disease is unclear. All mood stabilizers cause birth defects.

A. Lithium

Indications: (1) Mania

Buzz Words: T-wave flattening or inversion leading to U waves + bipolar disorder I → patient treated with lithium

Fetus with atrialization of right ventricle and decreased RV cardiac output → Ebstein anomaly 2/2 taking Li in first trimester of pregnancy

Bipolar patient + Li treatment + nonsteroidal antiinflammatory drug (NSAID; e.g., ibuprofen) treatment for knee pain + seizures, altered mental status, coma → Li toxicity 2/2 NSAID use

- **aspirin** and **sulindac** are the only NSAID or NSAID-like drugs that do not precipitate lithium toxicity
- treat Li toxicity with (1) fluid resuscitation, and (2) dialysis

<u>Mechanism</u>: Unknown

<u>Side Effects</u>: **Normal level side effects:** Diabetes insipidus, weight gain, N/V, tremor (Tx with propranolol), hypothyroidism, cardiac dysrhythmias, leukocytosis, GI irritation/cramps, Ebstein anomaly I in first trimester of pregnancy

Li intoxication: (1) Seizures, (2) altered mental status, and (3) coma, death

B. Carbamazepine

<u>Indications</u>: (1) Trigeminal neuralgia, (2) seizures, (3) REM behavior disorder/periodic movement disorder, (4) intermittent explosive disorder, (5) bipolar disorder (I or II), (6) cyclothymia, and (7) long-term treatment of withdrawal from sedative-hypnotics (like barbiturates or benzos)

Buzz Words:

- Bipolar disorder + agranulocytosis → likely 2/2 carbamazepine (monitor weekly if <2000 ANC; d/c med if <1000 ANC)
- Bipolar disorder + increased AFP in a 20 week pregnancy → neural tube defect 2/2 carbamazepine or valproate
- Bipolar disorder + Steven-Johnson syndrome (SJS) + East Asian
- Microcephaly + hypoplasia of distal phalanges of fingers + hypoplasia of toes + excess hair + cleft palate + hirsutism + rib anomalies → fetal hydantoin syndrome 2/2 carbamazepine or phenytoin use
- Sharp, severe shooting pain in face + bolt of lightning + brought on by touch + unshaven side of face with pain → tic douloureux (trigeminal neuralgia) → Tx with carbamazepine

<u>Mechanism</u>: (1) Sodium channel blocker but unknown how it modulates psychiatric disease

<u>Side Effects</u>: (1) Hyponatremia, (2) SJS in East Asians, (3) potent inducer of P450 system, (4) agranulocytosis, (5) craniofacial defects (fetal hydantoin syndrome), and (6) autoinducer that increases metabolism of drugs such as warfarin, phenytoin, and lamotrigine

C. Valproic Acid (aka Valproate)

<u>Indications</u>: (1) Generalized seizures, (2) intermittent explosive disorder, (3) PTSD, (4) bipolar disorder I,

---

FOR THE WARDS

Do not use lithium with (1) digoxin, (2) pregnancy, (3) myasthenia gravis, (4) diuretics, (5) MI, (6) severe renal disease.

FOR THE WARDS

For patients on or considering lithium treatment, check Cr, UA, CBC, pregnancy test, blood glucose and EKG.

FOR THE WARDS

Lithium level checked q4–8 weeks. Li level of 0.6–1.2 mg is therapeutic.

FOR THE WARDS

For patients on carbamazepine, check CBC for agranulocytosis q2weeks for first 2 months and then q3mo afterwards; also check LFT, BMP, and ECG.

(5) cyclothymia, (6) rapid cycling, and (7) long-term treatment of withdrawal from sedative-hypnotics (like barbiturates or benzos)

Buzz Words: Mom with bipolar disorder + baby with neural tube defect, craniofacial malformations, hydrocephalus → neural tube defect 2/2 valproic acid use

- Mom can PPx with 4 g folate
  spina bifida, cardiac defects, facial clefts, hypospadias, craniosynostosis, and limb defects, particularly radial aplasia → fetal valproate syndrome
  Bipolar disorder + increased AFP in a 20 week pregnancy → neural tube defect 2/2 carbamazepine or valproate
  Bipolar disorder + elevated LFTs + hepatitis → valproate toxicity

Mechanism: (1) Sodium channel blocker but unknown how it modulates psychiatric disease

Side Effects: (1) Pancreatitis, (2) hepatitis, (3) CBC abnormalities, (4) sedation, (5) weight gain, (6) hair loss, and (7) neural tube defect

D. Lamotrigine

Indications: (1) Depression stage of bipolar disorder, (2) epilepsy, (3) alcohol dependence, (4) binge eating disorder, (5) bulimia nervosa, (6) infantile spasms, (7) essential tremor, and (8) cluster headache

Buzz Words: Bipolar disorder + SJS. Likely 2/2 lamotrigine (less likely carbamazepine unless East Asian)

Mechanism: (1) Sodium channel blocker but unknown how it modulates psychiatric disease

Side Effects: (1) SJS, (2) leukopenia, (3) N/V/D, (4) hepatic failure

- avoid with OCPs; OCPs (drospirenone, ethinyl estradiol) will **lower** level of lamotrigine
- monitor leukopenia with CBC q6–12 months

E. Topiramate (e.g., Topamax)

Only drug where knowing the brand name (Topamax) is useful. Brand names will not be tested directly, but there is a brand name mnemonic you may find useful ("Dopa"max because topiramate makes patients confused, difficulty with memory, sedated)

Indications: (1) Migraine prophylaxis, (2) epilepsy, (3) alcohol dependence, (4) binge eating disorder (helps patient lose weight), (5) bulimia nervosa, (6) infantile spasms, (7) essential tremor, (8) cluster headache, and (9) migraine prophylaxis

Buzz Words: Alcohol abuse disorder + requires drug that reduces craving + patient not responsive to acamprosate, naltrexone → topiramate

Mechanism: (1) Sodium channel blocker, enhances GABA(A), antagonizes AMPA/kainite glutamate receptors, weakly inhibits carbonic anhydrase, but unknown how it modulates psychiatric disease

Side Effects: (1) SJS, (2) leukopenia, (3) N/V/D,; and (4) hepatic failure

- avoid with OCPs; OCPs (drospirenone, ethinyl estradiol) will **lower** the level of lamotrigine

Indications: (1) **Depression stage** of bipolar disorder, (2) epilepsy, (3) alcohol dependence, (4) binge eating disorder, (5) bulimia nervosa, (6) infantile spasms, (7) essential tremor, and (8) cluster headache

Buzz Words: Bipolar disorder + SJS. Likely 2/2 lamotrigine (less likely carbamazepine unless East Asian)

Mechanism: (1) Sodium channel blocker but unknown how it modulates psychiatric disease

Side Effects: (1) SJS, (2) leukopenia, (3) N/V/D, and (4) hepatic failure

- avoid with OCPs; OCPs (drospirenone, ethinyl estradiol) will **lower** the level of lamotrigine
- monitor leukopenia with CBC q6–12 months

Benzodiazepines

All benzos enhance GABA transmission, have anticonvulsant properties, decrease anxiety, and are metabolized in the liver by glucuronidation and oxidation EXCEPT for lorazepam. Oxazepam and temazepam are metabolized by **glucuronidation** ONLY

Examples: Shortest half life → alprazolam (Xanax) → highest risk of abuse

Short half life → midazolam, triazolam

Middle half-life → lorazepam → moderate risk of abuse
- lorazepam is equipotent in IM/PO/IV

Longest half-life → clonazepam (klonopin), low risk of abuse

Indications: (1) Alcohol withdrawal, and (2) anxiety disorders

Buzz Words: Alcohol abuse disorder + no alcohol >24 hours → benzos (e.g., lorazepam) to avoid alcohol withdrawal, delirium tremens

Patient with suicidal ideation + overdoses on benzos → treat with flumazenil

Mechanism: (1) Potentiate GABA, specific mechanism unclear

> **FOR THE WARDS**
> For topiramate, monitor leukopenia with CBC q6–12 months

> **MNEMONIC**
> Benzo withdrawal is deadly, along with Booze (alcohol) and Barbiturate withdrawal (the 3 B's)

Side Effects: **Toxicity**: (1) Miosis, (2) nystagmus, (3) somnolence, and (4) slurred speech

Withdrawal: (1) Same as alcohol, most notably delirium tremens → can lead to death, and (2) seizures

Psychotherapy

This section will briefly outline the types of psychotherapies you will be expected to know for the shelf. You will most likely need to explore each psychotherapy more in depth for your clerkship, but just make sure you know key buzzwords (e.g., dialectical behavioral therapy [DBT] → Tx for borderline personality disorder).

A. DBT

Indications: Borderline personality disorder

Description: **Individual component**: therapist and patient discuss issues on diary cards. It is necessary to keep suicidal urges or emotional issues from disrupting group sessions.

Group component: Group meets once weekly and learns to use specific skills categorized into four modules: (1) core mindfulness skills, (2) interpersonal effectiveness skills, (3) emotional regulation skills, and (4) distress tolerance skills.

B. Cognitive Behavioral Therapy (CBT)

Indications: Depression, anxiety

Description: Individual sessions that focus on challenging emotional response to maladaptive thoughts and using behavioral techniques (e.g., breathing). Requires patient to do homework.

C. Biofeedback

Indications: (1) Panic disorder, (2) migraines, (3) hypertension, (4) asthma, and (5) incontinence

Description: Modulation of physiological response through improving awareness of heart rate and blood pressure. A type of behavioral therapy.

D. Motivational Interviewing

Indications: (1) Substance use disorder

Description: Nonjudgmental sessions that acknowledge the difficulty of quitting the substance of abuse but focus on steps to take for change.

E. Parent Management Training

Indications: (1) Parents of a child with oppositional defiant disorder, and (2) parents of a child with conduct disorder

Description: Parent management training trains parents to manage their children's behavioral problems at school and at home. The focus is to utilize social learning techniques based upon operant conditioning to correct maladaptive parent-child interactions.

Behavioral Science and Ethics

Although patient characteristics associated with adherence can appear on the medicine, surgery, and family medicine shelf exams, they are particularly frequent on the psychiatry shelf. Learn what to do and what not to do in the following ethical scenarios. These concepts test your mastery of building the patient-doctor relationship, the strength of which is most closely related to patient adherence.

In general, think how your doctoring preceptor would respond and answer accordingly. The safest answer is usually correct.

A. Patient With Suicidal Ideation

Action: Assess the threat (e.g., detailed plan vs. passing thought); if the threat is serious (e.g., detailed plan, consistent suicidal ideation); make sure the patient is admitted to hospital voluntarily or involuntarily. Patients may be held involuntarily if they are a threat to self or others.

Avoid: Assuming the threat is not serious. The question stem may contain fillers to obfuscate the severity of SI admission.

B. Patient Non-Adherent to Treatment or Test

Action: Ask why the patient is non-adherent, and be respectful.

Avoid: Referring the patient to another physician.

C. Patient Nonadherent to Total Lifestyle Change, Behavior

Action: Ask about the patient's willingness to change their behavior. If a patient is not willing, then the provider cannot move on to the next step of why, and the issue needs to be addressed.

Avoid: Forcing the patient to change if they are not willing to; avoid scaring the patient. Remember, D.A.R.E. does not work.

D. Patient Who Is Seductive

Action: Set limits; define tolerable behavior; and see the patient with a chaperone.

Avoid: Refusing to care for the patient, asking open ended questions, referring patient to another physician, entering into relationship with patient (never the right answer).

E. Patient Who Is Angry

Action: NURSE: Name the emotion (e.g., "You appear angry."). Understand why, and thank the patient for sharing. Recognize what the patient is doing right. Show support for the patient. Explore the emotion.

Avoid: Taking the patient's anger personally.

F. Patient Who Is Sad and Tearful

Action: NURSE: Name the emotion (e.g., "You appear angry."). Understand why, and thank the patient for sharing. Recognize what the patient is doing right. Show support for the patient. Explore the emotion.

Avoid: Using patronizing statements such as "do not worry," rushing the patient, and stating "I understand." Instead, further explore the emotion to better understand where the patient is coming from.

G. Patient Who Complains About Another Doctor

Action: Recommend that the patient speak to the other doctor directly.

Avoid: Saying anything to disparage the other doctor, intervening with care unless there is an emergent need.

H. Patient Who Complains About You or Your Staff

Action: Verify the complaint, speak to the staff member who was named in the complaint.

Avoid: Blaming the patient, being defensive.

I. Patient to Whom You Need to Break Bad News

Action: SPIKES: Set up the patient encounter by making sure they are sitting in a chair with social support nearby. Ask about the patient's perception of what is going on. Ask the patient for an invitation or for permission to share the bad news. Explain your own knowledge of the bad news; make sure to preface by statements that convey the gravity of the situation (e.g., "I'm worried" or "I have bad news"). Manage the patient's emotion after the bad news is shared. Summarize the situation and suggest concrete next steps.

Avoid: Sharing bad news when the patient is in a vulnerable position (e.g., standing up while on the phone), breaking bad news without warning.

J. Patient Being Evaluated for Decision-Making Capacity

Action: Determine if the patient meets the criteria for being a legally competent decision maker, including (1) whether the patient is ≥18 or legally emancipated through marriage, military, or financial independence; (2) whether the patient makes and communicates a choice; (3) whether the patient knows and understands the benefit and risks; (4) whether the patient's decision is stable over time; (5) whether the patient's decision is congruent to their value system; and (6) whether the decision is not a result of a mood disorder, hallucinations, or delusions. Patients with adequate decision-making capacity can refuse labs, imaging (e.g., computed tomography [CT] scans) and treatment.

Avoid: Assuming the patient lacks decision-making capacity if less than 18 (remember marriage, military, and financial independence from parents).

K. Patient Who Is a Jehovah's Witness and Needs a Blood Transfusion

Action: Determine if the patient meets the criteria for not needing informed consent (e.g., legally incompetent, implied consent in an emergency with no ability for communication, patient waived the right to informed consent).

Avoid: Giving blood if the patient does not give consent, but does not meet one of the exceptions.

L. Patient With Meningitis Refusing Treatment

Action: Determine if the patient has a right to refuse treatment; in this case, the patient does not have a right because doing so would pose a threat to the health and welfare of others.

Avoid: Consulting hospital ethics committee unless there is a dilemma with no clear way to proceed.

M. Pediatric Patient With Nonemergent, Potentially Fatal Medical Condition, and Parents Refuse Treatment

Action: Seek a court order mandating treatment.

Avoid: Complying with parents' demand.
   Pediatric patient + nonemergent condition + no parental approval → proceed with treatment only after legal approval granted

QUICK TIPS
Pediatric patient + emergent condition + no parental approval → proceed with treatment anyway

N. Patient With HIV Diagnosis Refuses to Share With Significant Other

Action: Assess confidentiality rules; in this case, the significant other needs to be legally notified to prevent harm from transmission. Encourage the patient to discuss health and medical conditions with loved ones. Share patient results with the local health department.

Avoid: Allowing the patient to avoid disclosing a potentially fatal communicable disease.

GUNNER PRACTICE

1. A 78-year-old woman comes to the doctor with her husband because of difficulty sleeping during the past 12 months. Although she wakes up between 4 and 5 a.m. after going to bed at 10, she is unable to fall back asleep. She sometimes falls asleep during the day while reading a book. However, her day-to-day function is not impaired and her husband states that there have been no changes to her sleeping habits over this timeframe. She currently takes hydrochlorothiazide for hypertension that she states is well controlled, as well as metformin for diabetes mellitus. Her vital signs are blood pressure of 130/90, pulse of 75, respiratory rate of 12, temperature of 98.7°F, and oxygen saturation of 99% on room air. Physical examination notable for 1+ Achilles tendon reflex bilaterally. Patient is alert and oriented to name, place, and year. She states that she is in good spirits but is anxious about her sleep. Her affect is congruent to her stated mood. Mini-Mental State Examination (MMSE) is 29/30. When she asks what is wrong with her, what is the best way to respond?
   A. "I don't know. We need to gather more information and order some labs."
   B. "I don't know. We need to gather more information and order imaging of your head."
   C. "Rest assured, we will do everything we can to help and support you through this."
   D. "I don't know. We need to gather more information and order a sleep study."
   E. "Rest assured that what you are experiencing is normal."

2. A 54-year-old man with chronic schizophrenia comes to his psychiatrist for a routine follow-up appointment. He has been treated with haloperidol for the duration of his disease and is worried about the risk of EPS, such as tardive dyskinesia. He is currently not on medication for any other illness. Vital signs and physical exam are within normal limits. He is cooperative, speaks slowly with a regular rhythm, endorses a euthymic mood, and has a flat affect. No suicidal ideation, homicidal

ideation, auditory hallucinations, or visual hallucinations are reported. What is the most appropriate next step in treatment?

A. Decrease the dosage of haloperidol
B. Increase the time interval between each dose of haloperidol taken
C. Discontinue haloperidol
D. Switch from haloperidol to pimozide
E. Switch from haloperidol to aripiprazole
F. Switch from haloperidol to clozapine

3. A 47-year-old male with recently diagnosed schizophrenia presents to the emergency department with fever and altered mental status for the past 6 hours. The patient is accompanied by his spouse, who states that the patient works as a schoolteacher and has not had any recent ill contacts. She reports that he is generally healthy and only recently started taking a single medication. As far as she knows, he is up to date with his vaccines and had no recent or past head trauma. His vital signs show that he is febrile and tachycardic. His physical exam is noted for a rigid posture. His skin is warm to the touch. A CBC shows that the hemoglobin and hematocrit are normal, but the white blood cell count is high. The urine drug screen is negative. What is the most appropriate next step in management?

A. Order acetaminophen
B. Order cooling blankets
C. Discontinue his current medication regimen
D. Treat with ropinirole
E. Treat with dantrolene

ANSWERS: What Would Gunner Jess/Jim Do?

1. WWGJD? A 78-year-old woman comes to the doctor with her husband because of difficulty sleeping during the past 12 months. Although she wakes up between 4 and 5 a.m. after going to bed at 10, she is unable to fall back asleep. She sometimes falls asleep during the day while reading a book. However, her day-to-day function is not impaired and her husband states that there have been no changes to her sleeping habits over this timeframe. She currently takes hydrochlorothiazide for hypertension she states is well-controlled, as well as metformin for diabetes mellitus. Her vital signs are blood pressure of 130/90, pulse of 75, respiratory rate of 12, temperature of 98.7°F, and oxygen saturation of 99% on room air. Physical examination notable for 1+ Achilles tendon reflex bilaterally. Patient is alert and oriented to name, place, and year. She states that she is in good spirits but anxious about her sleep. Her affect is congruent to her stated mood. Mini-Mental State Examination is 29/30. When she asks what is wrong with her, what is the best way to respond?

Answer: E: "Rest assured, what you are experiencing is normal."

Explanation: There are two components to this question: (1) recognizing that this is normal aging, and (2) choosing how best to convey this to the patient. Sleep disturbance is part of the normal aging process. As folks grow older, total time spent in REM decreases and sleep becomes less efficient (e.g., higher proportion of stage 1 and 2 sleep). The National Board of Medical Examiners loves this type of normal aging question because it forces the examinee to read the whole question stem. Each clue here, from the 1+ Achilles tendon reflex to the 29/30 MMSE score is age-appropriate for our 78-year-old lady. This eliminates choices A, B, and D. That leaves two answer choices for how best to explain this phenomenon to the patient. C is not a great choice because it could imply that something is wrong with the patient and that she needs "help and support" outside of what is normal for her age. E is the best choice because the patient needs to hear that what she is going through is "normal."

A. "I don't know. We need to gather more information and order some labs." → Incorrect. Clues in the question stem point to a normal aging process. Labs are not needed for further evaluation.

B. "I don't know. We need to gather more information and order imaging of your head." →
Incorrect. Clues in the question stem point to a
normal aging process. Imaging is not needed for
further evaluation.

C. "Rest assured, we will do everything we can to
help and support you through this." → Incorrect.
The second sentence is too ambiguous and does
not explicitly state that the patient is experiencing a normal process of aging.

D. "I don't know. We need to gather more information and order a sleep study." → Incorrect. Clues
in the question stem point to a normal aging
process. A sleep study is not needed for further
evaluation. This may be an enticing answer if you
skimmed the question stem too fast. Make sure
to have "normal aging" near the top of your differential whenever you see a more than 65-year-
old patient in the question stem.

2. WWGJD? A 54-year-old man with chronic schizophrenia comes to his psychiatrist for a routine follow-up appointment. He has been treated with haloperidol for the
duration of his disease and is worried about the risk of
extrapyramidal symptoms, such as tardive dyskinesia.
He is currently not on medication for any other illness.
Vital signs and physical exam are within normal limits.
He is cooperative, speaks slowly with a regular rhythm,
endorses a euthymic mood, and has a flat affect. No
suicidal ideation, homicidal ideation, auditory hallucinations, or visual hallucinations are reported. What is the
most appropriate next step in treatment?

Answer: E: Switch from haloperidol to aripiprazole.

Explanation: This is a Tx/Mgmt question that tests
your understanding of antipsychotic side effects,
particularly with EPS. Remember that all antipsychotics present a risk of EPS, which includes
akathisia, acute dystonia, parkinsonism, and
tardive dyskinesia. Tardive dyskinesia, in particular, has effective treatment and appears after 4
months of antipsychotic use. The examinee has
to decide whether it is appropriate to decrease,
discontinue, or switch from haloperidol. For patients who suffer from schizophrenia, decreasing
the dose of the antipsychotic is rarely the correct
answer. Although a smaller dose decreases EPS
risk, there is an increased risk of recurrence of the
positive symptoms of schizophrenia. A, B, and

C can thus be ruled out. D–F offer alternatives to haloperidol. It is important to remember the side effect profile of antipsychotics. For instance, typicals have a higher EPS risk in general than atypicals. So pimozide, a high potency typical with a high risk of EPS, does not make sense as a replacement. Pimozide also prolongs QTc. Quickly rule out D. This leaves us with aripiprazole and clozapine—the latter of which can cause agranulocytosis, requires monitoring, and is considered a drug of last resort. Aripiprazole, on the other hand, has a much better side effect profile and is the correct alternative.

A. Decrease dosage of haloperidol → Incorrect. Reducing the dose of haloperidol may reduce the EPS risk, but would compromise the therapeutic effect and lead to hallucinations.

B. Increase the time interval between each dose of haloperidol taken → Incorrect. Increasing the time interval between each dose effectively reduces the concentration of haloperidol and would decrease the risk of EPS. However, this also increases the risk of the positive symptoms of schizophrenia.

C. Discontinue haloperidol → Incorrect. Discontinuing without an alternative is never the answer **unless** the patient's chief complaint is 2/2—an acute reaction from the drug.

D. Switch from haloperidol to pimozide → Incorrect. Pimozide is a high potency typical antipsychotic in the same group as haloperidol. High-potency typical antipsychotics have a high risk of EPS, although a lower risk of anti-HAM side effects. Pimozide is also known to prolong QTc.

F. Switch from haloperidol to clozapine → Incorrect. Clozapine is an atypical, but known as the atypical of last resort. While clozapine is the only atypical proven to reduce suicide risk, it has a nasty side effect profile, including agranulocytosis, seizures, hypotension, cardiomyopathy, and sialorrhea. Patients taking clozapine should get routine CBCs for monitoring.

3. WWGJD? A 47-year-old male with recently diagnosed schizophrenia presents to the emergency department with fever and altered mental status for the past 6 hours. The patient is accompanied by his spouse, who states the patient works as a schoolteacher and has not had

any recent ill contacts. She reports that he is generally healthy and only recently started taking medication. As far as she knows, he is up to date with his vaccines and had no recent or past head trauma. His vital signs show that he is **febrile and tachycardic. Physical exam** is noted for **a rigid posture.** His skin is warm to the touch. A complete blood count shows that the hemoglobin and hematocrit are normal but **white blood cell count is high.** Urine drug screen is negative. **What is the most appropriate next step in management?**

Answer: C: Discontinue haloperidol

Explanation: The patient has NMS, a deadly side effect of antipsychotics that can be discerned by the mnemonic FALTER: Fever, Altered mental status, Leukocytosis, Tremor, Elevated CPK, and Rigidity. The patient in this case had 4/6 symptoms (everything but tremor and elevated CPK). However, the key to this question is knowing the management steps, in the correct order, for NMS. For any question where medication is causing patient pathology, discontinue that medication immediately. The question stem masked the identity of the medication, but one could infer from the "recently diagnosed schizophrenia" that patient was taking an antipsychotic. Thus, C is the correct answer. After discontinuing the antipsychotic, supportive therapy, such as cooling blankets and acetaminophen, are next to reduce fever. Then dopamine agonists, such as ropinirole and dantrolene, are used to reverse the effects of the antipsychotic, which is a D2 receptor inhibitor.

A. Order acetaminophen → Incorrect. Acetaminophen can help reduce the patient's fever but does not take precedence over discontinuing the patient's medication. Supportive therapy is step #2.

B. Order cooling blankets → Incorrect. Cooling blankets can help reduce the patient's fever but does not take precedence over discontinuing the patient's medication. Supportive therapy is step #2.

D. Treat with ropinirole → Incorrect. Ropinirole can help treat NMS by reversing the effects of the D2 antagonist antipsychotics. However, it does not take precedence over discontinuing the culprit medication and supportive therapy to reduce fever. Dopamine agonist is step #3.

E. Treat with dantrolene → Incorrect. Dantrolene can help treat NMS by reversing the effects of the D2 antagonist antipsychotics. However, it does not take precedence over discontinuing the culprit medication and supportive therapy to reduce fever. Dopamine agonist is step #3.

Pediatric Psychiatry

Leo Wang, Hao-Hua Wu, and Olga Achildi

Pediatric psychiatry is organized into several subsections: adjustment disorders, eating disorders, incontinence, learning disorders, disruptive disorders, pervasive developmental disorders, genetic disorders, infectious diseases, and theories of development. This chapter encompasses a **lot** of information that spans everything from medicine to neurology. Luckily, pediatric psychiatry is so specialized that only a basic understanding of most of these diseases will be tested. As usual, focus on the **buzz words**, which will clue you in to recognizing the disease from the vignette. Upon recognizing a disease from the buzz words, the most important step in most diseases is diagnosis, treatment, and management. Prophylaxis rarely exists for many of these diseases and will be presented when relevant. Mechanisms of pediatric psychiatric diseases are even less well understood than adult psychiatric diseases, and as such are not often tested. In many cases, you will notice that parents are heavily involved in various aspects of each disease. This is because parents play a **major** role in many of these diseases, and fixing the disease in children often requires treating or managing both the child and parent together.

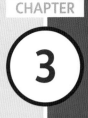

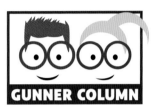

GUNNER COLUMN

Adjustment Disorders in Children

Adjustment disorders describe a group of symptoms that children can feel after a stressful life event because adequate coping mechanisms have yet to be developed. These include reactive attachment disorder, post-traumatic stress disorder (PTSD), acute stress disorder, and separation anxiety. These are highly tested on the psychiatric shelf, so you need to understand everything from the buzz words to the treatment/management for these disease processes.

A. Reactive Attachment Disorder of Infancy/Early Childhood

Buzz Words: Limited response to caregivers and others + limited positive affect + repeated changes in primary caregivers + **>9 months** + **<5 years** + episodes of irritability

Clinical Presentation:

Type I versus type II
- Cruel to animals, siblings, or other children
- Weak crying response
- No reciprocal smile response
- Often malnourished
- Tactile defensiveness

Type I = Inhibitory
- Do not respond in developmentally appropriate fashion to social interactions
- Hypervigilant, ambivalent, contradictory

Type II = Disinhibited
- Varied, indiscriminant attachments

PPx: Ensure children have safe and stable living situation with positive interactions with caregivers

MoD: Pathogenic care 2/2 one of the following:
- Persistent disregard for child's basic emotional needs
- Disregard of physical needs
- Repeated changes of primary caregiver
- Neglect (sensory deprivation) leads to brain abnormalities

Dx:
1. Rule out autism, depression, intellectual disability, adjustment disorder
2. Thorough psychiatric evaluation with assessment for episodes

Tx/Mgmt:
1. Individual and family counseling

B. PTSD in Children

Buzz Words: Major life stressor + separation anxiety + decreased sociability + avoidance/arousal symptoms occurring months/years after event + bed wetting + increased muscle tone/startle response + >1 month

Clinical Presentation: Children can get PTSD just like adults. In these situations, assess for the symptoms of PTSD, which include avoidance and arousal symptoms, occurring for longer than 1 month. Recognize that these symptoms, when occurring less than 1 month, are actually described by acute stress disorder.

PPx: Severity depends on parents' response to trauma as well

MoD: Increased catecholamine activity caused by dysregulation of hypothalamus-pituitary axis; prolonged sympathetic response with loss of self-regulation

Dx:
1. Psychiatric evaluation
2. Assess for the presence of 3+ of avoidance symptoms and 2+ arousal symptoms with sleep

disturbance, increased muscle tone, and startle response (Table 3.1)

Tx/Mgmt:
1. Cognitive behavioral therapy (CBT)
2. Psychological first aid (PFA) to teach problem-solving skills and calming
3. Eye movement desensitization and reprocessing (EMDR)
4. Play therapy

C. Acute Stress Disorder in Children

Buzz Words: Exposure to traumatic event + re-experiencing of event + numbing/detachment or depersonalization + amnesia + reduced awareness + **2 days–4 weeks**

Clinical Presentation: Acute stress disorder in children is the early equivalent of PTSD, taking place less than 4 weeks from a traumatic event . Children will often present with symptoms similar to adults, which include reexperiencing the event with numbing and detachment.

PPx: Parents' response to trauma affects severity

MoD: Thought to be precursor to PTSD

Dx:
1. Assess exposure to event in setting of avoidance and arousal symptoms for less than 1 month and longer than 2 days

Tx/Mgmt:
1. Cognitive behavioral therapy (CBT)—overcome denial/avoidance, teach coping
2. Selective serotonin reuptake inhibitor (SSRI)
3. Anticonvulsant
4. Problem-focused coping to control stressor (most effective unless stress or uncontrollable)
5. Emotion-focused coping (to reduce own arousal and distress)

D. Separation Anxiety Disorder

Buzz Words: Abdominal pain during school days or excessive fear of going to school + no physical symptoms

QUICK TIPS
80% of children burn victims will get this

QUICK TIPS
PTSD > 1 month, Acute Stress Disorder < 1 month

TABLE 3.1 Avoidance Versus Arousal Symptoms in PTSD

Avoidance Symptoms	Arousal Symptoms
Efforts to avoid thoughts, feelings related to event	Difficulty falling/staying asleep
Inability to recall aspect	Irritability or outburst of anger
Markedly diminished interest	Hypervigilance
Feeling detached or estranged	Exaggerated startle response
Restricted range of affect	
Sense of foreshortened future	

during the weekends/summers when child is with mother + refuses to sleep alone + **>4 weeks**

Clinical Presentation: This behavior is normal for patients that are 7–11 months old, and most patients diagnosed are between ages of 7–11 years old. Of patients between 7 and 11 years old, 5% will get this disorder. Parents are likely to have anxiety disorder.

PPx: Overprotective parents can precipitate separation anxiety

MoD: Often develops as coping mechanism to major life stressor

Dx:

1. Thorough psychiatric and medical evaluation

Tx/Mgmt:

1. CBT
2. SSRIs

Eating Disorders in Children

Eating disorders in children are characterized by a persistent failure to eat, decreased weight, an onset before the age of 6 with symptoms lasting for longer than 1 month. As a physician, an important point is to always rule out food insecurity.

A. Pica

Buzz Words: Eating of non-nutritive substances + >1 month

Clinical Presentation: Pica is present in 10%–30% children between the age of 1 and 6 years, and in one-quarter of institutionalized mentally retarded children. It is equally prevalent in boys and girls, and usually begins at age 1 or 2 years, remitting by adolescence in most cases. Some major complications of pica include poisoning, anemia, intestinal obstruction, and parasites.

PPx: N/A

MoD: Thought to be due to nutritional insufficiency or prenatal neglect

Dx:

1. Rule out anemia and other medical causes
   a. Schizophrenia
   b. Iron deficiency
   c. Zinc deficiency
   d. Kleine-Levin syndrome (sleep for weeks and wake up ravenously hungry)
2. Test for iron deficiency, check hemoglobin levels, iron, and zinc

Tx/Mgmt:
1. CBT
2. SSRIs

B. Rumination Disorder

Buzz Words: Repeated food regurgitation that is pleasurable, tension-relieving, or attention-seeking + failure to thrive + pain/nausea + bad breath + chapped lips + >1 month

Clinical Presentation: Rumination disorder is rare and most common in children from 3 months to 1 year, particularly in mentally retarded children; it is slightly more common in males and occurs in nervous and anxious individuals. Side effects include esophagitis, recurrent dental problems, excessive salivation, anemia, and social ostracism.

PPx: N/A

MoD: Thought to arise from physical illness or severe stress in the setting of parental neglect; may also be an attention-seeking behavior from the child

Dx:
1. Rule out medical causes including GERD and pyloric stenosis (projectile vomiting)
2. Review eating habits, observe infants during feeding

Tx/Mgmt:
1. Behavioral changes
   a. posture adjustments
   b. reducing feeding distractions
   c. encouraging parental attention
2. Psychotherapy
3. Operant procedures that structures patients with:
   a. "time out"
   b. electric shock
   c. pepper sauce, lemon juice on tongue
   d. overcorrection wash lips, use soap and lotion
   e. satiation, bring in food often

> **QUICK TIPS**
> Note that adults get rumination disorder, but will have normal weight and no pain/nausea

Incontinence in Children

A. Encopresis

Buzz Words: Involuntary or intentional passage of feces in inappropriate places + occurs once/month for 3+ months + **starts at age 4**

Clinical Presentation: This is a disease in which children pass feces in inappropriate places and occurs at least once a month for at least 3 months. Often times, these children are constipated because they do not use the bathroom enough and as a result defecate at inappropriate intervals. This is why stool softeners are great treatments for these patients. As a rule, encopresis must be diagnosed **after** age 4.

PPx: N/A

MoD: Often, this can be caused by a child not defecating for several days leading to constipation and the passage of stool at inappropriate times

Dx:
1. Check for fecal retention
2. Thorough medical and psychiatric evaluation

Tx/Mgmt:
1. Psychotherapy = behavioral modification that only rewards defecation
2. Stool softeners
3. Bowel catharsis

B. Enuresis

Buzz Words:

Urinating into bed or clothes + occurs 2/week for 3 months + >5 years old + causes marked impairment → Enuresis

Urinating into bed or clothes + occurs 2/week for 3 months + <5 years old + causes marked impairment → **Normal**

Clinical Presentation: This is a disease in which children void at inappropriate times or locations. There are two subtypes of enuresis. Primary enuresis occurs in patients who were never previously continent, and secondary enuresis occurs in patients after they were previously continent. This must occur in patients after the age of 5 and must occur at least twice a week for 3 months. Enuresis can further be classified by when it occurs; nocturnal enuresis occurs at night and diurnal enuresis occurs in the day. Remember, this process can be voluntary or involuntary.

If a patient presents with enuresis-like symptoms before the age of 5, he or she cannot be diagnosed yet by definition! This is a common question on the shelf (<5 years old vs. ≥5 years old).

PPx: N/A

MoD: Caused by a combination of anxiety, genetics, sleep apnea, structural abnormalities

Dx:
1. Urinalysis and urine culture
2. Rule out diuretic use
3. Rule out medical causes:
   a. DM
   b. seizures
   c. urethritis

Tx/Mgmt:
1. Behavioral training (shock, bell, alarm, and pad)
2. Imipramine (TCAs)
3. DDAVP (watch out for H_2O intoxication)
   a. headaches = main side effect
   b. nausea
   c. hyponatremia

Learning Disorders

Learning disorders include a subset of disorders regarding the ability for young children to understand and respond to information. The most commonly tested learning disorder is attention deficit disorder (ADD)/attention deficit hyperactivity disorder (ADHD)—for this, know everything from the buzzwords to the treatment/management. The single most important thing you can do for a patient with a learning disorder is to test their hearing and vision; this concept is important both in real life and on the psychiatry shelf.

A. ADHD
Buzz Words: Temper tantrum in preschool + difficult with peers in elementary + internal sense of restlessness as an adolescent + chronic disorganization as an adult + inattention and hyperactivity (easily distracted, careless mistakes, forgetful, difficulty listening, reluctance to put forth effort) + occurs in both school and home + <6 months + presentation before 7 years

Clinical Presentation: ADHD is 67% comorbid with Conduct and Oppositional Defiant Disorder (ODD) and these patients have a 25% chance of developing antisocial personality disorder (PD). This is a disease where genetics probably plays a key role, and remember these kids have low self-esteem. In 20%, these symptoms present out to adulthood.

PPx: Prevent alcohol exposure, tobacco exposure

MoD:
1. Likely dysregulation of NE and dopamine
2. Low norepinephrine and low dopamine levels
3. No dopamine in frontal lobe...all gas and no brakes

Dx:
1. Rule out hearing/vision problems
2. Complete medical history
3. Assess for six symptoms of attentiveness, hyperactivity, or both that **persist >6 months and present before 7 years old** that **occur in two settings (e.g., home + school)**

4. Inattentive symptoms
   a. careless mistakes
   b. difficulty with attention
   c. difficulty listening
   d. no instructions
   e. lack of organization
   f. reluctance to put forth effort
   g. losing things easily
   h. forgetful, easily distracted
5. Hyperactivity-impulsivity symptoms
   a. restlessness
   b. difficulty in quiet activities
   c. driven by a motor
   d. excessive talking
   e. blurts out answers (impulsive)
   f. doesn't wait turn (impulsive)

Tx/Mgmt:

1. Methylphenidate (Ritalin, Concerta, Metadate, Focalin)
   a. blocks dopamine (DA) reuptake
   b. upregulates DA
   c. side effects are that of stimulants
   d. can still be used if tics already there
2. Dextroamphetamine (Dexedrine, Dextrostat)
3. Amphetamine salts (Adderall)
   a. blocks DA **and** NE reuptake **and** stimulates release
   b. upregulates DA and Ne
   c. side effects are that of stimulants
4. Pemoline = stimulant drug
5. Atomoxetine
   a. non-stimulant, so it will NOT cause tics
   b. NE reuptake inhibitor so upregulates NE
   c. dry mouth, insomnia, decreased appetite side effects
      Indications
      • ADHD with substance abuse
      • ADHD with tics
      • ADHD with comorbid tics
6. Reboxetine
   a. nonstimulant
   b. NE reuptake inhibitor
   c. dry mouth, insomnia, decreased appetite side effects
7. SSRI adjunct
   • prevents NE reuptake and increases NE in synapse

8. If stimulants don't work, can try alpha-2 agonists like clonidine or guanfacine
   a. cause sedation
9. Psychotherapy
10. Parental counseling
11. Group therapy
12. Send patient to **therapeutic day school** if not working out at regular school

B. Learning Disorders, Not Otherwise Specified (NOS)

Buzz Words: Does not meet expected achievement for age, education, intelligence, and it is NOT due to organic cause

Clinical Presentation: Learning disorder NOS was recently renamed "Specific Learning Disorder," which is a catch-all term that now includes problems like dyslexia, dyscalculia, and more. Dyslexia is trouble with reading despite normal intelligence. Dyscalculia is trouble with math despite normal intelligence. Dysgraphia is trouble with writing despite normal intelligence. A rarer learning disorder is Language Processing Disorder, which is a condition in which children have trouble attaching meaning to the sounds that they hear.

PPx: None

MoD: None

Dx:

1. Rule out vision/hearing problems
2. Full medical exam including ruling out dyspraxia (difficulty in motor control)

Tx/Mgmt: Specific to type of learning disorder and is not commonly tested

C. Selective Mutism

Buzz Words: Children refuse to speak in certain situations only, but have normal language development lasting more than 1 month

Clinical Presentation: Selective mutism is typically thought of as an extension of social anxiety. This can also be present in adults. Patients with selective mutism refuse to speak in certain situations where speech would be expected, despite a complete understanding of speech and the ability to speak. Selective mutism is often perceived as shyness.

PPx: N/A

MoD: Inherited predisposition to anxiety with increased function in amygdala

QUICK TIPS
Dyspraxia is comorbid with many learning disorders

Dx:

1. Test language and speech
2. Rule out other problems affecting communication (autism, schizophrenia, ADHD)
3. Ensure symptoms occur only in specific setting, >1 month and affects function

Tx/Mgmt:

1. Psychotherapy
2. Behavioral therapy
3. Anxiety management
4. SSRIs

QUICK TIPS

Selective mutism, if left untreated, can cause chronic depression and anxiety

D. Tourette's Disorder

Buzz Words: Repetitive blinking, throat-clearing or licking + clearing throat or other vocal tic occurring many times a day + everyday + lasting longer than 1 year + <18 years old

Clinical Presentation: This is a disorder with motor and verbal tics in children <18 years old. Tourette's occurs in boys more often, and will usually begin at age 7.

PPx: Avoid stimulants

MoD:

1. Dopamine dysregulation in caudate and decreased GABA
2. Too much dopamine in the caudate and too little GABA in the caudate as well (GABA stuff per casefiles)
3. Fifty-percent concordance in monozygotic twins suggesting genetic predisposition

Dx:

1. Test for obsessive-compulsive disorder (OCD) and ADHD
2. Assess for:
   a. 2+ motor tics, 1+ vocal tics that occur many times a day, almost every day for >1 year **onset prior to age 18;** this must cause distress or impairment in social/occupational functioning

Tx/Mgmt:

1. Pimozide (DA receptor antagonist)
   a. causes QT prolongation
2. Haloperidol
3. Clonidine (activates presynaptic autoreceptors in locus coeruleus to decrease NE)
4. Guanfacine (activates presynaptic alpha-2 adrenergic receptor to decrease NE)

E. Mental Retardation

Buzz Words: Impaired disability in self-care, learning, mobility, receptive/expressive language in child <18 years old

Clinical Presentation: Mental retardation is infrequently tested on the pediatric psychiatry shelf and is a complicated umbrella term for many different pathologies. As such, the ability to recognize etiologies of mental retardation is typically sufficient.

PPx: N/A

MoD:

1. Organic/idiopathic
   - no discernable pathologic basis
   - comorbidities include
     - epilepsy
     - cerebral palsy
     - autism
     - fetal alcohol
     - down syndrome
   - men > women
   - higher in non-white
2. Prenatal (genetic)
   - Fragile X → 30%–50%
   - Down syndrome
   - TORCH infections
   - Prader-Willi (50%–70% paternal deletion)
   - chromosomal basis
3. Perinatal or postnatal (problems by 2 years)
   - alcohol related
   - anoxia
   - lead
   - mercury
   - associated with mom smoker

Dx:

1. Evaluate for hearing/vision
2. Thorough medical exam
3. IQ Test
4. Assess for disability in two areas, such as self-care, learning, mobility, receptive/expressive language, etc. (Table 3.2)

Tx/Mgmt: Not tested

Disruptive Disorders in Pediatric Psychiatry

Disruptive disorders are some of the most common problems faced by parents in pediatric psychiatry and as such are tested frequently on the shelf exam. As an organizing principle, remember that these disruptive disorders may induce a vicious cycle of behavior that leads to decreased positive interactions with the parent that

TABLE 3.2 Mental Retardation Severity

Severity	IQ	Characteristics	Function
Mild	50–70	Not detected until child is in school; child will complete elementary education	Can live/work independently; requires modest level of support
Moderate	35–50	Social isolation in elementary school	Requires high level of support, but can work independently in some capacity
Severe	20–35	Minimal speech; poor motor development	Requires extensive supervision
Profound	<20	Absent speech; absent motor skills	Constant supervision with nursing through life

IQ, Intelligent quotient.

further exacerbates the child's behavior. Thus, parenting plays a key role in the prophylaxis and mechanism of these disorders. Children with disruptive disorders often develop them secondary to violent disciplinary techniques in the context of a genetic predisposition. As a rule of thumb, treating these disorders involves parent training, and multimodal treatments that use school, family, and community resources to enforce behaviors and expectations, with infrequent use of medications, like antipsychotics or lithium, to limit aggressions.

A. Oppositional Defiant Disorder

Buzz Words: Hostile and defiant behavior + temper tantrums + arguments + deliberately annoying/trolling + blaming others + no violation of laws + occurring >6 months

Clinical Presentation: ODD is a disorder in which children are generally defiant towards authority, but importantly do not actually break any rules or laws. ODD is usually diagnosed at 3–8 years old and is highly associated with ADHD (50%). ODD can occasionally lead to conduct disorder, and is estimated to be in 5% of children.

PPx: Precipitated from parent and family environment; prevent violent discipline by parents

MoD: Thought to occur through a combination of genetics and parenting environment including violent disciplinary action

Dx:
1. Complete medical evaluation
2. Assess for frequency and intensity of hostile and aggressive behaviors occurring more than 6 months

Tx/Mgmt:
1. Psychotherapy (behavioral training)
2. Parenting skills training
3. Parental-child interaction therapy
4. Social skills training

B. Conduct Disorder

Buzz Words: Violation of social norms (destruction of property, theft) + significant impairment + <18 years old + >6 months

Clinical Presentation: Conduct disorder is the big brother of ODD and in some sense is more of an exaggerated version, where hostile and defiant behavior has evolved into actual violation of rules and laws. Of these patients, 40% will be diagnosed with antisocial PD. Conduct disorder is also highly comorbid with ADHD and substance abuse. Of note, children with conduct disorder can feel remorse about their actions; oppositely, children with conduct disorder who do not feel remorse often will later be diagnosed with antisocial PD.

PPx: Precipitated from parent and family environment

MoD: Thought to occur through a combination of genetics and parenting environment including violent disciplinary action; patients have serotonin dysfunction or **decreased 5-HIAA** in CSF

Dx:
1. Complete medical evaluation
2. Assess for frequency and intensity of hostile and aggressive behaviors occurring >6 months with violation of social norms and rules and causes significant impairment

Tx/Mgmt:
1. Multimodal
   a. firm rules, consistency
   b. psychotherapy on behavior
2. Antipsychotics and lithium for aggression
3. SSRI for impulsivity and aggression
4. Some patients enjoy psychodynamic therapy

QUICK TIPS

Subtypes are child-onset conduct disorder (<10) and adolescent-onset conduct disorder (10–17)

Pervasive Developmental Disorders

Pervasive developmental disorders include a spectrum of diseases that impair all aspects of development. On the shelf, you will be expected to recognize and differentiate between the pervasive developmental disorders, and thoroughly work up these patients. This includes medical, lab, psychological, physical testing, and speech and language evaluation. The most commonly tested developmental disorder is autism.

A. Autism Spectrum Disorder

Buzz Words: Social impairment + lack of interest + poor eye contact + stereotyped use of language or language delay + repetitive motor movements + preoccupations with objects

Clinical Presentation: The Autism Spectrum Disorder (ASD) is an umbrella term encompassing a lack of social function and communication with restricted behavior and interests. The term "Asperger's" used to encompass children with purely motor delays, but without delays in speech and development; however, it is now just categorized as a disease that falls within the spectrum. Of patients on the autism spectrum, 70% have comorbid mental retardation.

PPx: Eighteen-month screening for autism

MoD: Unknown

Dx:

1. Rule out (r/o) medical causes
    a. vision and hearing test
    b. acquire maternal age, health, alcohol use, smoking
    c. acquire gestation age, perinatal complications, NICU stays
    d. look for presence of infection, maternal diabetes, jaundice, birth defects
    e. look for neurologic problems
    f. look for cardiac problems
    g. test parents' IQ
2. Lab testing should include:
    a. **lead** levels → pica, ASD
    b. chromosomal analyses
    c. molecular-genetic
3. Psychological evaluation
    a. developmental progression
    b. intelligence
    c. behavioral observation scales
4. Physical evaluation
    a. somatic growth-height
    b. weight
    c. head circumference
5. Speech and language evaluation

Tx/Mgmt:
1. Behavioral and family interventions
2. Speech, occupational, and physical therapy
3. Community support, parent training

Criteria for Diagnosis of Autism

1. Assess for 6+ total symptoms from social interaction impairment, social communication problem, and restrictive behavior/interests
2. Social interaction impairment (2+)
   a. impairment of nonverbal behavior such as poor eye contact
   b. failure to develop peer relationships
   c. lack of spontaneous seeking to share enjoyment
3. Social communication problem (1+)
   a. stereotyped use of language
   b. language delay (if no language delay or cognitive delay, question suggests Asperger's)
   c. lack of varied or spontaneous play
4. Restrictive behavior/interests (1+)
   a. intense preoccupation with object
   b. inflexible adherence to rules
   c. repetitive motor movements

B. Rett Disorder (Cerebroatrophic Hyperammonemia)

Buzz Words: Decreased head circumference **growth rate** during 5–48 months + loss of previously acquired hand skills + loss of social interaction + impaired language, psychomotor development + stereotyped hand movements + cyanosis + seizures + GI problems + occurring at 5 months only in females

Clinical Presentation: Rett disorder is caused by an abnormality on the X-chromosome and is associated with the MECP2 gene. It is a disease that only girls can get. The most common findings include small head, hands, and feet, and repetitive hand movements. Rett's was recently removed from the DSM and is more often categorized as a neurologic disorder. Of note, the previous name of Rett syndrome, cerebroatrophic hyperammonemia, has nothing to do with the disease itself, and high ammonia levels were an incidental finding.

PPx: Screen females who were normal for the first 5 months of life and started deteriorating

MoD: Associated with the **MECP2 gene** on X-chromosome

Dx:
1. R/o medical causes
   a. **vision** and **hearing** test
   b. acquire maternal age, health, alcohol use, smoking

    c. acquire gestation age, perinatal complications, NICU stays
    d. look for presence of infection, maternal diabetes, jaundice, birth defects
    e. look for neurologic problems
    f. look for cardiac problems
    g. test parents' IQ
    h. rule out Angelman syndrome, cerebral palsy, autism
  2. Lab testing should include:
    a. **lead** levels
    b. chromosomal analyses
    c. molecular-genetic
  3. Psychological evaluation
    a. developmental progression
    b. intelligence
    c. behavioral observation scales
  4. Physical evaluation
    a. somatic growth-height
    b. weight
    c. head circumference
  5. Speech and language evaluation

Tx/Mgmt:
  1. Physical therapy/hydrotherapy
  2. Occupational therapy
  3. Speech-language therapy
  4. Feeding assistance
  5. Medications for seizures, cardiac abnormalities

C. Childhood Disintegrative Disorder (Heller Syndrome)

Buzz Words: Loss of language and social skills (bladder/bowel control, ability to play) + impaired social interactions + stereotyped behaviors or stereotyped interests + typically beginning at age 2 but before age 10

Clinical Presentation: This is the male equivalent of Rett disorder. Childhood Disintegrative Disorder leads to the loss of language skills and social functioning with stereotyped interests and behaviors between the ages of 2 and 10. Although females can get it, 80% of those with Childhood Disintegrative Disorder are males.

PPx: N/A

MoD: Can be precipitated by various conditions, including lipid storage diseases, subacute sclerosing panencephalitis, tuberous sclerosis, and leukodystrophy

Dx:
  1. Rule out medical causes
    a. vision and hearing test
    b. acquire maternal age, health, alcohol use, smoking

    c. acquire gestation age, perinatal complications, NICU stays

    d. look for presence of infection, maternal diabetes, jaundice, birth defects

    e. look for neurologic problems

    f. look for cardiac problems

    g. test parents' IQ

2. Lab testing should include:
   a. lead levels
   b. chromosomal analyses
   c. molecular-genetic
3. Psychological evaluation
   a. developmental progression
   b. intelligence
   c. behavioral observation scales
4. Physical evaluation
   a. somatic growth-height
   b. weight
   c. head circumference
5. Speech and language evaluation

Tx/Mgmt:
1. Behavioral therapy
2. Environmental therapy
3. Antipsychotics/antiepileptics

Genetic Disorders

Genetic disorders are tested on the psychiatry shelf but are rarely managed by psychiatrists in real life. As such, recognizing these diseases and understanding their mechanisms will be the extent to which you will be tested on the psychiatry shelf. Here, focus specifically on the buzz words above all else. Other important physician's tasks, if relevant, will be provided.

A. Prader-Willi Syndrome
Buzz Words: Mental retardation + obesity 2/2 hyperphagia "eats compulsively" + hypogonadism + almond shaped eyes + skin picking + hypotonia + aggression, argumentative + narrow face

MoD: (1) Chromosome 15 paternal deletion (can be boy or girl)

B. Angelman's Syndrome
Buzz Words: Seizures + strabismus → heterotopia → eyes are not properly aligned with one another + sociable with episodic laughter

MoD: Deletion on maternal chromosome 15

> **MNEMONIC**
> The 3 S's: seizures, strabismus, sociable

C. Fragile X

Buzz Words: Eleven-year-old developmental delay, poor school and social performance, 50 IQ with macrocephaly + long face + macroorchidism + autistic + delayed speech + "flapping hands"

Clinical Presentation: Complications:

- seizures
- mitral valve prolapse (MVP)
- dilation of the aorta
- tremor
- ataxia
- ADHD-like behavior
- Fragile X is the most common cause of inherited mental retardation

MoD:

- X-linked dominant
- CGG repeats with anticipation

D. Down Syndrome

Buzz Words: Simian crease + big tongue + white spots on iris + decreased tone + oblique palpebral fissures + epicanthal folds

Clinical Presentation:

1. Mild-moderate mental retardation
2. Speech delay
3. Gross motor delay
   - difficulty hopping on one foot
   - low percentile for height and weight
4. Fine motor delay

Medical Cx:

1. Cardiac
   a. Ventricular septal defect (VSD)
      - 2/6 murmur
2. Endocardial defects (more common)
2. Gastrointestinal
   a. Hirschsprung's
   b. Intestinal atresia
   c. Imperforate anus
   d. Annular pancreas
3. Endocrine
   a. Hypothyroidism
4. Musculoskeletal (MSK)
   a. Atlanto-axial instability
5. Neuro
   a. Increased risk of Alzheimer's by 30–35 (APP is on chromosome 21)
6. Cancer
   a. 10× increased risk of ALL

E. Neurofibromatosis 1
Buzz Words: Café-au-lait spots + seizures + large head
MoD: Autosomal dominant

F. Hurler Syndrome
Buzz Words: Mucopolysaccharide defect + coarse facies + short stature + cloudy cornea
MoD: Autosomal recessive

G. Smith-Magenis Syndrome
Buzz Words: Broad, square face + short stature (like Hurler syndrome) + self-injurious (like Cornelia de Lange)
MoD: Deletion on chromosome 17

H. Williams Syndrome
Buzz Words: Elfin-appearance + friendly + increased empathy and verbal reasoning ability
MoD: Chromosome 7

I. Fetal Alcohol Syndrome
Buzz Words: ADHD-like symptoms + microcephaly (vs. fragile X, which has macrocephaly) + smooth philtrum + mental retardation (most common acquired cause)

J. Congenital Cytomegalovirus Infection
Buzz Words: Seizures + chorioretinitis + hearing impairment + periventricular calcifications → in the brain + petechiae at birth + hepatitis

K. Congenital Rubella Syndrome
Buzz Words: Seizures + hearing impairments + cloudy cornea/retinitis + heart defects + low birth weight

L. Cerebral Palsy From Birth Asphyxia
Buzz Words: Abnormal muscle tone + unsteady gait + seizures + mental retardation + learning disability

M. Cornelia de Lange Syndrome
Buzz Words: Intrauterine growth restriction + hypertonia + distinctive facies + limb malformation + self-injurious behavior + hyperactive

N. CHARGE Syndrome
Buzz Words:
Coloboma of the eye (hole in one of the structures of the eye)
Heart defects
Atresia of the nasal choanae (back of nasal passage)

MNEMONIC
ugly name so wants to kill self, restricted in womb, limb malformation after suicide attempt

Cornelia De Lange

Retardation of growth and development
Genital and/or urinary abnormalities
Ear abnormalities and deafness
MoD: Abnormality on chromosome 8

O. DiGeorge Syndrome (aka 22q11.2 Deletion Syndrome)
Buzz Words: Autism spectrum + heart disease + palate defects + hypoplastic thymus + hypocalcemia
MoD: Chromosome 22 deletion

P. Maple Syrup Urine Disease
Buzz Words: Vomiting + seizures + lethargy + coma + acidosis with stress + illness + neurological damage

Infectious Diseases in Pediatric Psychiatry

A. Pediatric Autoimmune Neuropsychiatric Disorders Associated With Streptococcal Infections (PANDAS)
Buzz Words: Patient who was recently "sick" with strep-related infection presents with **OCD** symptoms and **tics**
Clinical Presentation: There is only a single disease related to pediatric infections and psychiatry and that is PANDAS. Recognize that strep infections can lead to OCD and tic symptoms in children. This is the extent to which you will be tested on this process.
PPx: N/A
MoD: N/A
Dx:
1. Antistreptolysin O (ASO) titer rises 3–6 weeks post infection
2. Antistreptococcal DNAaseB (AntiDNAse-B) titer rises 6–8 weeks postinfection

Tx/Mgmt:
1. IVIG
2. Plasma exchange
3. Antibiotics
4. SSRIs + CBT for OCD
5. **Risperidone for tics**

Theories of Development

The theories of psychosocial development are infrequently tested on the psychiatry exam (Table 3.3). In short, these theories have essentially broken down child development into phases that are characterized by discrete changes and behaviors. These theories are not

TABLE 3.3 Theories of Development

	Erikson Psychosocial Development Stages	Piaget Cognitive Development Stages	Freud Psychosexual Stages
0–1	Trust vs. mistrust	Sensorimotor—child explores world through sensory and motor contact; objective permanence and separation anxiety develop	Oral—focus of libido is mouth, tongue, lips, breast feeding
1–3	Autonomy vs. shame		Anal—major development in toilet training, children experiment with urine and feces
3–5	Initiative vs. guilt	Preoperational—child uses words and images but cannot logically reason; is egocentric	Phallic—develop and resolve Oedipus complex
5–11	Industry vs. inferiority	Concrete operational—child thinks about objects in concrete fashion; death is permanent	Latent—none, children develop superego
11–Adolescence	Identity vs. role diffusion	Formal operational—think abstractly; deductive reasoning; hypothetical thinking	Genital—reaching sexual maturity
21–40	Intimacy vs. isolation	—	—
40–65	Generativity vs. stagnation	—	—
>65	Integrity vs. despair	—	—

explicitly tested on the shelf, but some of these terms may be brought up in the occasional question stem. This material is more helpful for clinics. Feel free to skip this subsection if pressed for time.

99 AR

Erikson Stages of Development

GUNNER PRACTICE

1. A 14-year-old boy is brought to your office by his mother due to complaints that he is becoming increasingly "frustrating" at school. According to his teachers, he has become irritable and uncooperative over the past few years in the classroom setting. At home, he refuses to wash the dishes and recently declined to take out the trash. He has repeated several years of elementary school, and is frequently turning in assignments late, if at all. His IQ test is within normal limits. He is at the 75th percentile for height and 60th percentile for weight. During exam, the patient is cooperative but sarcastic. Which of the following is the most likely diagnosis?
   A. Normal adolescent behavior
   B. Conduct disorder
   C. Oppositional defiant disorder
   D. ADHD
   E. Reading disorder

2. An 8-year-old boy presents to your office after complaints of impulsivity and excessive motor activity over the past year. His friends describe him as the "class clown." Physical examination and lab studies show no abnormalities and he is prescribed methylphenidate. Which of the following is comorbid with this patient's condition?
   A. Adjustment Disorder
   B. ASD
   C. Separation Anxiety Disorder
   D. Learning Disability
   E. Conduct Disorder

3. A 14-year-old girl is brought to her physician because of difficulty making friends at school. Recently, she has become increasingly frustrated that she has to go to school because she does not want to talk to others. On exam, she is quiet and polite but serious. She is in the 50th percentile for height and weight for her age with a normal IQ. When you ask her why she does not want to go to school, she is concerned that her "voice is changing." Upon further questioning, you later learn she has skipped school for the last week and spent her time at a local library instead. Which of the following is the most likely diagnosis?
   A. ADHD, inattentive type
   B. Social phobia
   C. Selective mutism
   D. Autistic disorder
   E. Normal adolescent behavior

Notes

ANSWERS: What Would Gunner Jess/Jim Do?

1. WWGJD? A 14-year-old boy is brought to your office by his mother due to complaints that he is becoming increasingly "frustrating" at school. According to his teachers, he has become irritable and uncooperative over the past few years in the classroom setting. At home, he refuses to wash the dishes and recently declined to take out the trash. He has repeated several years of elementary school, and is frequently turning in assignments late, if at all. His IQ test is within normal limits. He is at the 75th percentile for height and 60th percentile for weight. During exam, the patient is cooperative but sarcastic. Which of the following is the most likely diagnosis?

Answer: C, Oppositional defiant disorder

Explanation: This is a classic presentation of oppositional defiant disorder, where a child is difficult to deal with and does not respond to authority, leading to decline in functioning in school (hence turning assignments in late, repeating school years). Importantly, this must occur in the setting of normal IQ and development. Keep in mind that this patient does not disobey any laws and therefore cannot be thought to have conduct disorder.

- A. Normal adolescent behavior → Incorrect. Where, to some extent, normal adolescent behavior can lead to defiance, the impaired functioning as a result of this makes ODD a much more likely possibility.
- B. Conduct disorder → Incorrect. Conduct disorder would require violations of laws (theft, graffiti, etc.)
- D. ADHD → incorrect. ADHD does not explain his refusing to wash dishes at home and take out trash. Irritability and defiance are not characteristic of ADHD.
- E. Reading disorder → Incorrect. Reading disorder, or dyslexia, may lead him to turn in assignments late but does not explain the other symptoms.

2. WWGJD? An 8-year-old boy presents to your office after complaints of impulsivity and excessive motor activity over the past year. His friends describe him as the "class clown." Physical examination and lab studies show no abnormalities and he is prescribed methylphenidate. Which of the following is comorbid with this patient's condition?

Answer: D, Learning disability

Explanation: Excessive impulsivity and motor activity is usually characterized by ADHD, and frequently these children are labeled the "class clown." ADHD is comorbid with learning disabilities.

A. Adjustment Disorder → Incorrect. There is no association between ADHD and Adjustment Disorder.

B. ASD → Incorrect. There is no association between ADHD and autism.

C. Separation Anxiety Disorder → Incorrect. There is no association between ADHD and Separation Anxiety Disorder.

E. Conduct Disorder → Incorrect. There is an association between ADHD and Conduct Disorder but ADHD is almost ALWAYS comorbid with learning disability.

3. WWGJD? A 14-year-old girl is brought to her physician because of difficulty making friends at school. Recently, she has become increasingly frustrated she has to go to school because she does not want to talk to others. On exam, she is quiet and polite but serious. She is in the 50th percentile for height and weight for her age with normal IQ. When you ask her why she does not want to go to school, she is concerned that her "voice is changing." Upon further questioning, you later learn she has skipped school for the last week and spent her time at a local library instead. Which of the following is the most likely diagnosis?

Answer: B, Social phobia

Explanation: Young, adolescent girls often have changes through puberty that they can feel embarrassed about, leading to social phobia, or social anxiety disorder. The fear of being scrutinized or judged by others leads to her not wanting to speak publicly or go to school.

A. ADHD, inattentive type → Incorrect. She has no symptoms of inattention or hyperactivity.

C. Selective mutism → Incorrect. Although selective mutism is comorbid with social anxiety disorder, selective mutism leads to an absolute refusal to communicate in a specific scenario. Instead, she does not enjoy going to school altogether. She also has not met the 1 month criteria.

D. Autistic disorder → Incorrect. She has normal communication abilities on exam.

E. Normal adolescent behavior → Incorrect. Normal adolescents may feel embarrassed about puberty changes, but the decline in function (her not attending at school) indicates a psychiatric problem.

Substance-Related Disorders

Anup Bhattacharya, Hao-Hua Wu, Leo Wang, and Olga Achildi

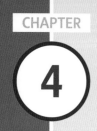

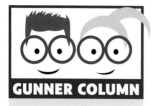

GUNNER COLUMN

Introduction

Having a firm understanding of substance-related disorders is a key component towards doing well on the psychiatry shelf. Learn the buzz words and treatment for both toxicity and withdrawal for each drug.

Substance-related disorders are conditions that result from acute intoxication, abuse, and dependence (now collectively known as "substance use"), and/or withdrawal from a variety of substances, which will be covered in this chapter.

Some key overarching facts that provide immediate high-yield benefit for the psychiatry shelf include the following.

First, the three drugs that are deadly in withdrawal are the "3 B's": benzodiazepines, barbiturates, and booze (alcohol).

Second, diseases caused by substance abuse are high yield because they can show up on multiple shelf exams. Wernicke encephalopathy and Korsakoff syndrome, for example, will serve you well, not only for psychiatry but also for neurology and medicine.

Regarding the four physician tasks for the chapter, you will not have to worry about Prophylaxis (PPx) as that would simply be avoidance of the substance itself. However, Mechanism of Disease (MoD), Diagnostic Steps (Dx), and Treatment/Management (Tx/Mgmt) are frequently tested. The Tx/Mgmt algorithm for toxicity, withdrawal, and dependence of each substance is different, but use the following "Gunner Column" pro-tip regarding intoxication versus withdrawal to organize your study. The chapter is organized by substance-induced disease states and each disorder includes Buzz Words, PPx, MoD, Dx, and Tx/Mgmt. Clinical Presentation is left blank when Buzz Words provide enough clues to recognize the disease state in a question stem.

QUICK TIPS

Intoxication vs. Withdrawal.

In general, the physiologic effects of a particular substance's intoxication vs. withdrawal will be the opposite of each other. For example, alcohol and other depressants slow the body down, with reduced blood pressure and heart rate, while withdrawal from these same substances can cause increased blood pressure and heart rate.

Substance Use Disorder (DSM-V)

The psychiatry shelf has transitioned to wider usage of *Diagnostic and Statistical Manual of Mental Disorders,* fifth edition (DSM-V) and will continue to replace questions requiring knowledge of prior criteria. DSM-V does not use *substance abuse* or *substance dependence.* Instead, a new term, *substance use disorder,* has been employed and is characterized by two or more of the following occurring within a 12-month period:

1. The substance is often taken in larger amounts or over a longer period than was intended.
2. There is a persistent desire or unsuccessful effort to cut down or control the use of the substance.
3. A great deal of time is spent in activities necessary to obtain the substance, use the substance, or recover from its effects.
4. Craving, or a strong desire or urge to use the substance.
5. Recurrent use of the substance resulting in a failure to fulfill major role obligations at work, school, or home.
6. Continued use of the substance despite having persistent or recurrent social or interpersonal problems caused or exacerbated by the effects of its use.
7. Important social, occupational, or recreational activities are given up or reduced because of use of the substance.
8. Recurrent use of the substance in situations in which it is physically hazardous.
9. Use of the substance is continued despite knowledge of having a persistent or recurrent physical or psychological problem that is likely to have been caused or exacerbated by the substance.
10. Tolerance, as defined by either of the following:
    a. A need for markedly increased amounts of the substance to achieve intoxication or desired effect.
    b. A markedly diminished effect with continued use of the same amount of the substance.
11. Withdrawal, as manifested by either of the following:
    a. The characteristic withdrawal syndrome for that substance (as specified in the DSM-V for each substance).
    b. The substance (or a closely related substance) is taken to relieve or avoid withdrawal symptoms.

Alcohol Intoxication

Buzz Words: Disinhibition + slurred speech + ataxia + vomiting + euphoria

Clinical Presentation: N/A

PPx: N/A

MoD: Activates GABA receptors (which are inhibitory) and inhibits glutamate activity (which normally is excitatory) → net effect is central nervous system (CNS) depression

Dx:
1. Blood alcohol content
2. Gamma glutamyl transferase (GGT)
3. Carbohydrate-deficient transferrin

Tx/Mgmt:
1. Thiamine (to PPx Wernicke's)
2. Supportive (fluids)
3. Gastric lavage

Tx/Mgmt for Alcohol Use Disorder: (1) Alcoholics anonymous, (2) Naltrexone (mu opioid receptor antagonist), (3) Disulfiram (acetaldehyde dehydrogenase inhibitor that can lead to flushing, headache, nausea/vomiting), (4) Acamprosate, (5) Topiramate (reduces alcohol cravings)

Alcohol Withdrawal

Buzz Words: Tremors + autonomic hyperactivity including HTN and tachycardia + insomnia + anxiety + nausea + vomiting + seizures + hallucinations (visual and tactile) + delirium

Clinical Presentation:

Alcoholic hallucinosis: Occurs 1–2 days after last drink and is predominantly characterized by visual hallucinations. Many question stems present patients who have a history of alcoholism and are suddenly hospitalized often for an unrelated problem. Within a few hours of their hospital stay, they start experiencing severe withdrawal, which can often start with visual hallucinations (alcoholic hallucinosis) but can become something even more severe: delirium tremens (DTs).

Delirium tremens: Occurs 2–4 days after the last drink and is predominantly characterized by autonomic hyperactivity symptoms, including—but not limited to—tremors, tachycardia, and seizures. If not treated appropriately with benzodiazepines, it can be deadly.

PPx: N/A

MoD: Disinhibition of GABA receptors (which are ordinarily inhibitory) → net effect is CNS excitation

Dx:
1. CIWA scale

Tx/Mgmt:
1. Benzos (lorazepam, oxazepam, temazepam, chlordiazepoxide)
2. Magnesium for seizures

Wernicke-Korsakoff Syndrome

Buzz Words:
Altered mental status + ophthalmoplegia + ataxia (AOA) → Wernicke encephalopathy
Confabulation + amnesia + psychomotor agitation (CAP) + mammillary body atrophy → Korsakoff syndrome
Clinical Presentation: N/A
PPx: (1) Ensure adequate body thiamine stores
MoD: Thiamine deficiency
Dx:
1. Based on clinical features, as described in "Buzz Words"
Tx/Mgmt:
1. For Wernicke's, replenish thiamine before glucose and consider supportive therapy (fluids)
2. For Korsakoff syndrome, damage is irreversible

Video on Delirium Tremens

Tobacco Abuse

Buzz Words: Nausea + vomiting + hypersalivation + hypertension + tachycardia + ataxia + headaches + dizziness + sweating + abdominal discomfort → tobacco intoxication
Clinical Presentation: N/A
PPx: N/A
MoD: Nicotine is the major chemically active substance in tobacco. Nicotine binds to (aptly named) nicotinic Ach (nAch) receptors, which are ligand gated ion channels
Dx:
1. Patient history
Tx/Mgmt: N/A
Tx/Mgmt for Tobacco Use Disorder: (1) Nicotine replacement therapy (NRT), includes US Food and Drug Administration (FDA) approved nicotine gum/lozenges and transdermal patch; (2) Varenicline, which mimics the action of nicotine, is FDA approved for smoking cessation; (3) Bupropion, an antidepressant, is also FDA approved for smoking cessation → depressed patient with trouble quitting smoking gets bupropion

FOR THE WARDS
Important convention is pack-years, which is the number of packs smoked per day (on average), multiplied by the number of years smoked. For example, a person who has smoked 2 packs/day for 15 years, has a 30-pack-year smoking history.

QUICK TIPS
NEVER prescribe bupropion to an anorexic patient or a patient with a seizure history!

Tobacco Withdrawal

Buzz Words: Anxiety + irritability + depression + insomnia + difficulty concentrating + weight gain → tobacco withdrawal

Clinical Presentation: N/A

PPx: N/A

MoD: Disinhibition of nAch receptor

Dx:

1. Made clinically, with symptoms as described above, along with patient history

Tx/Mgmt:

1. NRT, includes FDA-approved nicotine gum/lozenges and transdermal patch
2. Varenicline

Marijuana Intoxication

Buzz Words: Dry mouth + impaired short-term memory + impaired motor skills and perception + red eyes

Clinical Presentation: N/A

PPx: N/A

MoD: Tetrahydrocannabinol (THC), the active ingredient in marijuana, actively binds the cannabinoid receptors

Dx:

1. Urine drug screen (UDS)

Tx/Mgmt: N/A

Tx/Mgmt for Marijuana Use Disorder: (1) Cognitive behavioral therapy (CBT); (2) motivational therapy

Marijuana Withdrawal

Buzz Words: N/A

Clinical Presentation: No physiological withdrawal effects

PPx: N/A

MoD: N/A

Dx: N/A

Tx/Mgmt: N/A

LSD Intoxication

Buzz Words: **Not violent** + depersonalization + derealization + illusions + hallucinations + synesthesias, pupillary dilation + tachycardia + diaphoresis + palpitations + tremors + "out of this world" experience + flashbacks

Clinical Presentation: N/A

PPx: N/A

MoD: Modulation of serotonergic activity in the brain

Dx:
1. Patient history/exam
Tx/Mgmt:
1. Supportive care and discontinuation of other serotonergic drugs to avoid serotonin syndrome
2. Use of cyproheptadine (serotonin receptor agonist) for serotonin syndrome
3. Gastric decontamination (in most serious of circumstances)
Tx/Mgmt for LSD Use Disorder: (1) CBT; (2) motivational therapy

gg AR
Video on Psychedelic Experience

LSD Withdrawal

Buzz Words: N/A
Clinical Presentation: No physiological withdrawal effects
PPx: N/A
MoD: N/A
Dx: N/A
Tx/Mgmt: N/A

MDMA Intoxication

Buzz Words: Illusions + hallucinations + pupillary dilation + tachycardia + diaphoresis + palpitations + tremors + hyperthermia + dance club raves
Clinical Presentation: N/A
PPx: N/A
MoD: Upregulates serotonin, dopamine, and noradrenaline release
Dx:
1. UDS
Tx/Mgmt:
1. Supportive care and discontinuation of other serotonergic drugs to avoid serotonin syndrome
2. Use of cyproheptadine for serotonin syndrome
3. Monitoring for hyperthermia, dehydration, seizures
4. Gastric decontamination in serious circumstances
Tx/Mgmt for MDMA Use Disorder: (1) CBT; (2) motivational therapy

FOR THE WARDS
MDMA is also known as "ecstasy" or "molly"

MDMA Withdrawal

Buzz Words: Depression + anxiety + confusion + fatigue + paranoia + loss of appetite + difficulty concentrating
Clinical Presentation: N/A
PPx: N/A
MoD: N/A

Dx:

1. Patient history

Tx/Mgmt:

1. Supportive care (maintaining fluids, as appropriate)

Inhalant Intoxication

Buzz Words: Adolescent experimenting with drugs + sniffing + belligerence + impaired judgment + drowsiness + agitation

Clinical Presentation: N/A

PPx: N/A

MoD: Various, unknown effects on both the CNS and the peripheral nervous system

Dx:

1. Patient history/exam

Tx/Mgmt:

1. Supportive care (maintain hydration)
2. Monitor vital signs

Tx/Mgmt for Inhalant Use Disorder: (1) CBT, (2) dialectical behavioral therapy, (3) biofeedback, (4) family therapy

Inhalant Withdrawal

Buzz Words: Nausea + muscle cramps + convulsions + sweating

Clinical Presentation: N/A

PPx: N/A

MoD: Various, unknown

Dx:

1. Patient history/exam

Tx/Mgmt:

1. Supportive therapy

Opioid Intoxication

Buzz Words: Miosis + constipation + drowsiness + nausea/vomiting + respiratory depression

Clinical Presentation: N/A

PPx: N/A

MoD: Act as agonists at mu opioid receptors in the brain

Dx: UDS, per patient history

Tx/Mgmt: Naloxone or naltrexone (opioid antagonists) as well as respiratory support to maintain ventilation

Tx/Mgmt for Opioid Use Disorder: (1) Methadone is used for opioid maintenance therapy for recovering addicts and it is

QUICK TIPS

Inhalants can cause encephalopathy!

QUICK TIPS

Tolerance does not develop to opioid miosis or constipation!

QUICK TIPS

Meperidine (Demerol) does not cause miosis on intoxication! Watch for serotonin syndrome with use of meperidine and other serotonergic agents.

QUICK TIPS

Many heroin addicts have a past history of receiving an opioid pain medication (oxycodone, morphine) prescribed by their physicians for severe pain. Over time, they had difficulty weaning off the opioid medication and became addicted to cheaper substances, such as heroin, to obtain their fix. This is yet another reason to be wary of prescribing opioid pain medications to your patients, unless absolutely necessary, particularly in the primary care setting!

long acting. Some side effects to watch for with methadone include QT interval prolongation; (2) Buprenorphine is another agent often used for recovering heroin addicts, and it serves as a partial opioid agonist that generally comes in the form of Suboxone, which is buprenorphine with naloxone, to prevent diversion of this treatment

Opioid Withdrawal

Buzz Words: Insomnia + rhinorrhea + yawning + sweating + piloerection + dilated pupils + hypertension + tachycardia + myalgia
Clinical Presentation: N/A
PPx: N/A
MoD: Disinhibition of activity at mu opioid receptor
Dx:
1. Patient history/exam
Tx/Mgmt:
1. Methadone (taper or maintenance therapy)
2. Buprenorphine
3. Clonidine often used for reduction of anxiety, muscle aches, and cramping

Benzodiazepine Intoxication

Buzz Words: Confusion + drowsiness + ataxia + incoordination + hypotension + impaired judgment + nystagmus + coma
Clinical Presentation: N/A
PPx: N/A
MoD: Increase the frequency of chloride channel opening for the GABA receptor
Dx:
1. UDS, per patient history
Tx/Mgmt:
1. Gradual weaning/detox of benzodiazepine from system, depending on initial level
2. **Flumazenil**, which is a benzodiazepine receptor antagonist
3. Supportive management
Tx/Mgmt for Benzodiazepine Use Disorder: (1) CBT; (2) group therapy

FOR THE WARDS
Although flumazenil is the answer on the shelf for benzo intoxication, the use of flumazenil is limited in practice to avoid seizures

QUICK TIPS
GHB is often used in narcoleptic patients, and it has received recognition as the "date-rape" drug.

QUICK TIPS
Alcohol and sedatives potentiate each other's effects and the combination of the two also can be deadly as both involve modulation of the same GABA receptor.

Benzodiazepine Withdrawal

Buzz Words: Sleep disturbances + anxiety + tremor + sweating + difficult concentrating + palpitations + hallucinations + seizures + psychosis + autonomic hyperactivity + death

Clinical Presentation: N/A
PPx: N/A
MoD: Disinhibition of activity of GABA receptor
Dx:
1. Patient history/exam
Tx/Mgmt: Similar to that for alcohol withdrawal:
1. Benzos
2. Magnesium for seizures

Barbiturate Intoxication

Buzz Words: Fluctuating levels of consciousness + drowsiness + shallow breathing + loss of coordination + sluggishness + respiratory distress in high doses
Clinical Presentation: N/A
PPx: N/A
MoD: Increase the duration of chloride channel opening for the GABA receptor
Dx:
1. UDS
Tx/Mgmt:
1. Maintain adequate ventilation and watch for respiratory depression, apply supplemental oxygen as needed
2. Supportive management
Tx/Mgmt for Barbiturate Use Disorder: (1) CBT, (2) group therapy

Barbiturate Withdrawal

Buzz Words: Restlessness + insomnia + nausea + vomiting + sweating + anxiety
Clinical Presentation: N/A
PPx: N/A
MoD: Disinhibition of activity of GABA receptor
Dx:
1. Patient history/exam
Tx/Mgmt:
1. Watch for autonomic hyperactivity and maintain supportive treatment

Non-Benzodiazepine Sedative Hypnotics Intoxication

Buzz Words: Sedation + sluggishness + no history of benzo/barbiturate/booze use
Clinical Presentation: N/A
PPx: N/A
MoD: Modulate chloride channel activity on GABA receptor

Dx:
1. Per patient history
Tx/Mgmt:
1. Supportive care
Tx/Mgmt for Non-Benzodiazepine Sedative Hypnotic Use Disorder:
   (1) CBT

Non-benzodiazepine Sedative Hypnotics Withdrawal

Buzz Words: Insomnia + anxiety + history of sedative/hypnotics use
Clinical Presentation: N/A
PPx: N/A
MoD: Disinhibition of activity of GABA receptor
Dx:
1. Patient history
Tx/Mgmt:
1. Supportive care mainly (withdrawal not as serious as benzodiazepine or barbiturate withdrawal)

Cocaine Intoxication

Buzz Words: Young adult + chest pain + dilated pupils + choreiform movements + excitability + psychosis
Clinical Presentation: N/A
PPx: N/A
MoD: Blocks re-uptake of dopamine and norepinephrine from the presynaptic terminal of the synapse so the concentration of these two neurotransmitters in the synaptic cleft is increased
Dx:
1. UDS
Tx/Mgmt:
1. Benzodiazepines to reduce autonomic hyperactivity
Tx/Mgmt for Cocaine Use Disorder: (1) Cocaine Anonymous and other group therapy; (2) motivational therapy; (3) CBT

Cocaine Withdrawal

Buzz Words: Depression + fatigue + lethargy + history of cocaine use
Clinical Presentation: N/A
PPx: N/A
MoD: Reduced concentrations of dopamine and norepinephrine in synaptic cleft
Dx:
1. Patient history/exam

QUICK TIPS
Never prescribe beta blockers to patients in acute cocaine intoxication because that will lead to unopposed alpha agonist and severe hypertension!

QUICK TIPS
Cocaine overdose is associated with cardiac arrhythmias.

QUICK TIPS
If you determine psychosis to be present in a teenager out of the blue, always suspect acute stimulant intoxication, and your next step in management, after ensuring the ABCs are secure, is to take a UDS!

Tx/Mgmt:
1. Supportive care

Methamphetamine Intoxication

Buzz Words: (Similar to acute cocaine intoxication, except without chest pain.) Young adult + dilated pupils + excitability + substance-induced psychosis

Clinical Presentation: N/A

PPx: N/A

MoD: Reverses direction of catecholamine transporter, leading to increased concentration and activity of catecholamines on their respective downstream targets

Dx:
1. UDS, per patient history

Tx/Mgmt:
1. Benzodiazepines to reduce autonomic hyperactivity

Tx/Mgmt for Methamphetamine Use Disorder: (1) 12-step support; (2) family intervention; (3) individual counseling

Methamphetamine Withdrawal

Buzz Words: Fatigue + depression + hunger + constricted pupils + history of stimulant use

Clinical Presentation: N/A

PPx: N/A

MoD: Reduced concentrations of dopamine and norepinephrine in synaptic cleft

Dx:
1. Patient history

Tx/Mgmt:
1. Supportive care

Phencyclidine Intoxication

Buzz Words: Rotatory nystagmus + **belligerent behavior** + ataxia + hypertension + autonomic hyperactivity + muscle rigidity + depersonalization + hallucinations

Clinical Presentation: Very high-yield on the shelf because its presentation mimics LSD intoxication. Violent patients likely have phencyclidine (PCP) intoxication, whereas nonviolent patients likely have LSD intoxication.

PPx: N/A

MoD: N-Methyl-D-aspartate (NMDA) receptor antagonist

Dx:
1. UDS

Tx/Mgmt:

1. Benzodiazepines to reduce autonomic hyperactivity
2. Haldol to manage acute belligerent behavior

Tx/Mgmt for PCP Use Disorder: N/A

Phencyclidine Withdrawal

Buzz Words: N/A

Clinical Presentation: No physiological withdrawal symptoms

PPx: N/A

MoD: N/A

Dx: N/A

Tx/Mgmt: N/A

Bath Salts Intoxication

Buzz Words: Autonomic hyperactivity + altered mental status + violent behavior + paranoia

Clinical Presentation: N/A

PPx: N/A

MoD: Multiple modulation of neurotransmitter networks, often serotonergic in origin

Dx:
1. Patient history

Tx/Mgmt:
1. Monitoring of acute changes in vitals
2. Supportive treatment

Tx/Mgmt for Bath Salt Use Disorder: N/A

Bath Salts Withdrawal

Buzz Words: N/A

Clinical Presentation: No physiological withdrawal symptoms

PPx: N/A

MoD: N/A

Dx: N/A

Tx/Mgmt: N/A

Polysubstance Abuse Intoxication

Buzz Words: Use history to determine the likelihood of polysubstance abuse.

Clinical Presentation: Polysubstance abuse refers to the consumption of more than one drug over a particular time period and the physiological and psychological consequences of such drug consumption. When considering the effects of multiple drugs on the physiological system, one needs to understand the mechanism of action

QUICK TIPS

Acute PCP intoxication can present with psychosis. Pay particular attention to the context of such a presentation. The time frame of symptom onset, the age of the patient, and the activities performed prior to presentation to a provider are clues that may help distinguish between drug intoxication with PCP and the first break of a schizophrenic patient.

99 AR

Showing Acute PCP Intoxication

QUICK TIPS

The use of psychoactive bath salts (PABS) has been steadily increasing with more frequent presentation of patients acutely intoxicated on these salts to the Emergency Department. The severity of acute intoxication can warrant care in the ICU setting.

of each particular drug, so that drugs that may act synergistically (i.e., alcohol and benzodiazepines) will, for example, have an effect that is more than the sum of each individually.

Common substances that are abused together are the following: (1) alcohol, tobacco, and marijuana; (2) various amphetamines; and (3) various prescription pain killers (narcotics).

Beyond this, this topic is unlikely to be tested in any further detail on the shelf exam.

PPx: N/A

MoD: Variable, dependent upon abused substances

Dx:

1. Patient history

Tx/Mgmt:

1. Variable, dependent upon abused substances

Tx/Mgmt for Polysubstance Abuse Disorder: (1) Variable, dependent upon abused substances

GUNNER PRACTICE

1. A 37-year-old male with a past medical history significant for chronic back pain is brought to the emergency department (ED) by his wife who found him unconscious on the living room floor. In the ED he is found with constricted pupils and is breathing with a respiratory rate of 6. Which of the following best represents his PCO_2 on presentation?
   A. 20
   B. 30
   C. 35
   D. 40
   E. 50

2. A 68-year-old alcoholic male is hospitalized for community-acquired pneumonia. One day after admission he complains of seeing things out of the ordinary that neither his physicians nor nurses can see. What would be the next best step in management?
   A. Flumazenil
   B. Naloxone
   C. Naltrexone
   D. Lorazepam
   E. Diazepam

3. A 29-year-old train driver crashes his train carrying 208 passengers. Fortunately, all on board survive with only minor injuries, but investigations reveal that the driver failed to appropriately react to a speed change prior to

jumping track. Hospital records reveal that the driver presented with memory loss and red eyes. What substance is likely to have been ingested by the conductor?

A. LSD
B. Cocaine
C. Marijuana
D. Alprazolam
E. Methamphetamine

ANSWERS: What Would Gunner Jess/Jim Do?

1. WWGJD? A 37-year-old male with a past medical history significant for **chronic back pain is** brought to the ED by his wife who found him **unconscious** on the living room floor. In the ED he is found with **constricted pupils** and is breathing with a **respiratory rate of 6.** Which of the following best represents his PCO_2 on presentation?

Answer: E, 50

Explanation: This patient is in acute opioid toxicity. He presumably uses opioids for treatment of his chronic back pain. Some buzzwords for opioid toxicity include constricted pupils and reduced respiratory rate. Since this patient is hypoventilating, we would expect this individual's PCO_2 to rise above the normal value of 40.

A. 20 → Incorrect. This represents alveolar hyperventilation.

B. 30 → Incorrect. This represents alveolar hyperventilation.

C. 35 → Incorrect. This represents alveolar hyperventilation.

D. 40 → Incorrect. This represents no change in ventilatory status.

2. WWGJD? A 68-year-old alcoholic male is hospitalized for community-acquired pneumonia. One day after admission he complains of **seeing things** out the ordinary that neither his physicians nor nurses can see. What would be the next best step in management?

Answer: D, Lorazepam

Explanation: This patient is in alcohol withdrawal and is experiencing alcoholic visual hallucinosis, an early sign. Benzodiazepines (specifically, lorazepam, oxazepam, and temazepam [LOT]) are preferred to manage withdrawal.

A. Flumazenil → Incorrect. This would be given in a benzodiazepine overdose.

B. Naloxone → Incorrect. This would be given in an acute opioid overdose.

C. Naltrexone → Incorrect. This is an opioid antagonist.

E. Diazepam → Incorrect. Only LOT benzodiazepines or chlordiazepoxide is used to treat alcohol withdrawal.

3. WWGJD? A 29-year-old train driver crashes his train carrying 208 passengers. Fortunately, all on board survive with only minor injuries, but investigations reveal

that the driver failed to appropriately react to a speed change prior to jumping track. Hospital records reveal that the driver presented with memory loss and red eyes. What substance is likely to have been ingested by the driver?

Answer: C, Marijuana

Explanation: This patient has memory loss, red eyes, and most importantly delayed reflexes from marijuana ingestion.

A. LSD → Incorrect. This would result in hallucinations but not red eyes with memory loss.

B. Cocaine → Incorrect. This would result in hyper-excitability and psychosis, but not red eyes with memory loss.

D. Alprazolam → Incorrect. This would result in sedation, not red eyes with memory loss.

E. Methamphetamine → Incorrect. This would result in dilated pupils and psychosis but not red eyes with memory loss.

Schizophrenia and Other Psychotic Disorders

James Janopaul-Naylor, Hao-Hua Wu, Leo Wang, and Olga Achildi

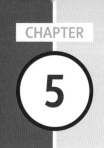

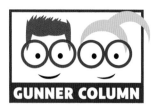

GUNNER COLUMN

Introduction

Psychosis is the term for a mental state that is disconnected from reality. Psychotic disorders can occur as a primary disease state that is subdivided by the length of symptoms or as a secondary aspect to the effects of a substance or another medical or psychiatric disease. Understanding the time course and minor symptoms that differentiate the different forms of psychosis is a quick way to score points on the shelf.

The basis for psychosis is poorly understood, but thought to be secondary to serotonin and dopamine dysfunction. As such, the current medications generally target those two neurotransmitter systems. In doing so, they cause a variety of unintended side effects, ranging from dry mouth to life-threatening neuroleptic malignant syndrome. Learning the main side effects of the different antipsychotics, and how to treat them, are incredibly high yield.

This chapter begins with describing the primary psychotic syndromes before discussing psychosis in the context of general medical conditions or secondary to medications or other drugs. As always, each disease process will be put into the four physician tasks the shelf exam will test you on: (1) Prophylactic (PPx) management, (2) Mechanism of Disease (MoD), (3) Stem Clues Establishing a Diagnosis, and (4) Treatment/Management (Tx/Mgmt). For the psychiatry shelf, pay particular attention to diagnosis and treatment.

A. Schizophrenia (>6 Months)

Buzz Words: Hallucinations (auditory and/or visual) + delusions + flat affect. Disorganized thinking + loses focus + enlarged ventricles + intact memory + **>6 months**

Clinical Presentation: Patients are aged 15–30 years for initial presentation, but can be older with known diagnosis. More common in men than women. Patient's chief complaint is a decline in function and social withdrawal (prodrome) or perceptual disturbances (Table 5.1), delusions, and disorganized thought process (psychotic). Can have 50% concordance rate in

TABLE 5.1 Perceptual Disturbances

Illusion	Misinterpretation of a real external sensory stimulus (e.g., interpreting a shadow as a dog)
Auditory hallucination	Common in schizophrenia. Command hallucinations tell patients to do something, and they put patients at a much higher risk of suicide
Visual hallucinations	More common in delirium and drug intoxications than schizophrenia. As opposed to illusions, visual hallucinations are completely novel images
Olfactory hallucinations	Often associated with a migraine aura or seizure
Tactile hallucinations	Can occur in drug abuse (usually cocaine), alcohol withdrawal, or benzodiazepine withdrawal. Formication is the specific feeling of insects crawling all over your skin

identical twins. Social history indicates patient was normal until high school, when he/she became more secluded and grades worsened. Alcohol, marijuana, and cocaine abuse is very common. Patient's mental status is any combination of delusions, hallucinations, disorganized speech, grossly disorganized behavior, agitation, or negative symptoms (flat affect, alogia, avolition).

PPx: None

MoD: Increased dopamine (D2 receptor) in the mesolimbic tract (positive symptoms) and decreased dopamine (D1 receptor) in the prefrontal cortex (negative symptoms). Other neurotransmitters may be involved

Dx:
1. History and mental status exam (MSE)
2. Urine drug screen (UDS), especially if symptoms are episodic in nature
3. Rule out a medical cause, such as recent steroid use, electrolyte imbalance (get a BMP), or thyroid dysfunction (TSH with T4)

Tx/Mgmt:
1. Antipsychotics for acute treatment (Table 5.2)
2. Hospitalization
3. Assess suicide risk by either seeing if they can contact for safety or assigning a 1-to-1
4. When counseling family for how they can help, using psychoeducation and encouraging them to minimize stress and conflict at home are the best options

MNEMONIC
The 5 A's of schizophrenia = anhedonia, avolition (apathy), alogia (poverty of speech), affect (flat), and attention (poor)

99 AR
Video that points out various diagnostic criteria with real patients

99 AR
Image with brief overview of Dopamine pathways

99 AR
Video of dopamine pathways

TABLE 5.2 Antipsychotic Medications

Antipsychotic	Mechanism of Action	Side Effects
Typical (e.g., haloperidol)	D2 dopamine receptor blockade primarily in the mesolimbic system. Greater anticholinergic side effects than atypicals	Nigrostriatal blockade (extrapyramidal symptoms) and anticholinergic effects. Overdoses can cause Neuroleptic Malignant Syndrome: "lead pipe" rigidity, high fever, elevated CPK, high blood pressure, tachycardia, and leukocytosis. Administer dantrolene, stop all antipsychotic medication, and actively cool the patient
Atypical (e.g., olanzapine, risperidone, quetiapine)	D2 dopamine receptor blockade in the mesolimbic and mesocortical. 5-HT$_{2A}$ serotonin receptor blockade	Serotonin blockade, tuberoinfundibular blockade (especially risperidone), less severe anticholinergic effects, and almost no nigrostriatal blockade
Clozapine (most effective antipsychotic)	D2 dopamine receptor blockade in the mesolimbic and mesocortical system. 5-HT$_{2A}$ serotonin receptor blockade	Agranulocytosis, hepatic failure, weight gain. Need to check complete blood count every 2 weeks. Also has same side effects as other atypicals, such as metabolic syndrome from serotonin blockade

B. Schizophreniform Disorder (1–6 Months)

Buzz Words: Hallucinations (auditory and/or visual) + delusions + flat affect. Disorganized thinking + loses focus + enlarged ventricles + intact memory + **1–6 months**

Clinical Presentation: Same clinical presentation as schizophrenia, except that in schizophreniform the symptoms are present for at least 1 month and no more than 6 months

PPx: None

MoD: See schizophrenia

Dx:

1. See schizophrenia

Tx/Mgmt:
1. The first step is a limited, 3- to 6-month course of antipsychotics (as opposed to indefinite treatment in schizophrenia). The next step is hospitalization

C. Brief Psychotic Disorder (<1 Month)

Buzz Words: Less than 1 month of symptoms + recent stressful life events such as immigration or post-partum + no substance use

Clinical Presentation: No history of other psychotic episodes or mood episodes. On the same spectrum as schizophreniform and schizophrenia; the only difference is the duration of symptoms.

PPx: None

MoD: Uncertain, but presumably decreased serotonin activity and excess dopamine (Table 5.3)

Dx:
1. See schizophrenia

Tx/Mgmt:
1. Atypical antipsychotic for 1–3 months
2. Education and reassurance
3. Monitor for recurrence

> **FOR THE WARDS**
> To impress on rounds (though less helpful for the shelf), point out that roughly 50%–80% of those with brief psychotic disorder will fully recover.

D. Delusional Disorder (>1 Month)

Buzz Words: See Table 5.4

Clinical Presentation: A delusion is defined as a fixed belief in a falsehood. However, the patient is still able to **work normally** or complete activities of daily living. Diagnostic criteria include a non-bizarre, fixed delusion for at least 1 month with no impairment in daily functioning.

PPx: None

MoD: Unknown

Dx:
1. History and MSE

Tx/Mgmt:
1. Psychotherapy
2. Selective serotonin reuptake inhibitor (SSRI) for anxiety and mood symptoms

E. Schizoaffective Disorder (Mood Episodes Plus >6 Months Psychosis)

Buzz Words: Depression (>2 weeks) or mania (>1 week) + hallucinations + delusions + >6 months (Table 5.5)

Clinical Presentation: Patient age can range from 15 to 50 years old with women more commonly affected than men. The chief complaint is a psychotic episode with a superimposed manic or depressed episode.

TABLE 5.3 Pathways Involved in Psychotic Disorders and Antipsychotics

Mesolimbic pathway	A dopamine pathway primarily involving the VTA and the nucleus accumbens. Plays a role in psychological reward and is responsible for the positive symptoms of schizophrenia
Mesocortical pathway	A dopamine pathway involving the VTA and its cortical projections. Plays a role in cognition and executive function, and is responsible for the negative symptoms of schizophrenia
Nigrostriatal pathway	A dopamine pathway involving the substantia nigra, caudate, and putamen. Plays a role in purposeful movement, and its blockade is responsible for extrapyramidal symptoms of treatment, such as parkinsonism, tremors, akathisia, and tardive dyskinesia
Tuberoinfundibular pathway	A dopamine pathway involving the hypothalamus and infundibular region, which is responsible for tonically inhibiting prolactin release. Antipsychotic treatment prevents this, disinhibiting prolactin and leading to galactorrhea, amenorrhea, and gynecomastia
Anticholinergic pathway	Antipsychotics, especially first-generation ones, inhibit the cholinergic system leading to dry mouth, constipation, dry eyes, blurred vision, drowsiness, and sedation
Serotonin pathway	Second-generation antipsychotics (atypicals) inhibit the serotonin pathway, often leading to sedation and weight gain

VTA, Ventral tegmental area.

PPx: None

MoD: Similar to schizophrenia, the major mechanism is thought to be serotonin and dopamine dysregulation

Dx:
1. History and MSE
2. UDS

Tx/Mgmt:
1. Treat current symptoms; that is, if they present with mania then provide mood stabilizers, or if they present with psychosis treat with antipsychotics
2. Manic and psychotic patients will require hospitalization
3. In patients refractory to antidepressants, mood stabilizers, and/or antipsychotics, electroconvulsive therapy is appropriate

TABLE 5.4 Types of Delusions

Persecutory delusions	Fear that "people" or the government is out to get them, or that they are being stalked or spied upon
Ideas of reference	Belief that a newspaper, television, radio, politician, or celebrity has a special message only intended for them
Delusions of grandeur	Belief that the person himself or herself is greater or more influential than they are
Somatic delusions	Belief that something is wrong with their body. Can include tactile hallucinations
Erotomanic or jealousy delusions	Belief that someone is in love with them or belief that their spouse or partner is unfaithful
Induced delusions	Sometimes called folie à deux, induced delusions occur when one person in a close relationship influences the other to adopt the same delusion. Treatment is to separate the two

TABLE 5.5 Differences Among Words With the "Schizo-" Prefix

Schizophrenia	Lifelong psychotic disorder, >6 months
Schizophreniform	Schizophrenia for <6 months
Brief psychotic disorder	Psychosis for <1 month, post-stressful event
Schizoaffective	Psychotic periods and mood disorder periods
Schizotypal	Paranoid personality with odd, magical, or eccentric beliefs
Schizoid	Withdrawn personality with lack of enjoyment from social interaction

F. Psychotic Disorder Secondary to a General Medical Condition

Buzz Words: Psychosis + "past medical history of" or "recent diagnosis of"

Clinical Presentation: Can occur at any age with a chief complaint of hallucinations, delusions, or disorganized thinking (Table 5.6).

PPx: Prophylactic treatment for the underlying condition as needed

MoD: Varies per condition

TABLE 5.6 Medical Conditions That Cause Psychosis

Central nervous system disease	Cerebrovascular (stroke or transient ischemic attack), multiple sclerosis, brain tumors, Huntington's, Alzheimer's, Parkinson's/Lewy body dementia, tertiary syphilis, epilepsy, encephalitis, and Creutzfeldt-Jakob disease
Endocrine disease:	Addison's, Cushing, hyperthyroid, hypothyroid, hypercalcemia, hypocalcemia, and hypopituitarism
Vitamin deficiency	Folate, niacin, and B12
Rheumatic disease	Systemic lupus erythematous and temporal arteritis
Hematologic disease	Porphyria

QUICK TIPS

The shelf will try to make it very clear if there is an underlying medical condition. Your main goal is to either diagnose it or pick the first appropriate treatment for that condition. If you think the psychosis is due to a medical condition do NOT treat with antipsychotics.

Dx:

1. Work up the medical condition (e.g., if signs and symptoms of thyroid dysfunction then order TSH). The shelf will try to make it clear which organ is affected, and your job will be to either pick the appropriate diagnostic test or treatment. For example, if you think it's lupus, get an anti-nuclear antibody (ANA) or treat with steroids (the shelf will not dive into details of the disease, e.g., ANA vs. anti-dsDNA, but rather will ask ANA vs. echocardiogram)

Tx/Mgmt:

1. Treat the underlying condition
2. If the symptoms persist despite resolution of the medical condition, then reevaluate for a primary psychiatric disorder

G. Substance-Induced Psychosis

Buzz Words:

Multiple people needed to restrain + nystagmus → phencyclidine (PCP) psychosis

Dilated eyes, agitated, tachycardia → cocaine and PCP psychosis

Visual hallucinations for several hours + nonviolent → lysergic acid diethylamide (LSD) psychosis

Recently changed medication regimen or recently started a new medication + psychosis → medication induced psychosis

Clinical Presentation: Common drugs that cause substance-induced psychosis are stimulants (e.g., cocaine) and hallucinogens, such as LSD and PCP. It can also be induced by medications such as steroids.

PPx: Avoid future use of same medication

MoD: Alters dopaminergic and serotonergic neurotransmission. PCP blocks the *N*-methyl-ᴅ-aspartate (NMDA) receptor. LSD and ecstasy activate serotonin receptors. Common causes of substance-induced psychosis include the following:

Medications: corticosteroids, levodopa, anticonvulsants, antihistamine, anticholinergics, beta blockers, digitalis, fluoroquinolones, and methylphenidate (all stimulants)

Drugs: alcohol, cocaine, LSD, ecstasy, marijuana, benzodiazepines, barbiturates, and PCP

Dx:
1. Patient history and MSE

Tx/Mgmt:
1. If a patient is agitated and a danger to others, physical restraints or chemical sedation (haloperidol and lorazepam)
2. Remove the offending causative agent (e.g., steroids)
3. If the patient is not agitated, but is distressed by the hallucinations, reassurance is appropriate.

99 AR

Differential diagnosis of delusions

GUNNER PRACTICE

1. A 28-year-old man is brought to the hospital by police after he was found wandering on the railroad tracks. He appears malnourished and unkempt. Although he agrees to be interviewed, he often loses focus and will often stare at the wall for a few seconds and then laugh. He has no known medical history, but per a contacted family member he was hospitalized in a psychiatric institution when he was 19 for similar symptoms. He doesn't remember any of the meds he has ever taken. A urine toxicology screen and blood alcohol level are negative. A decision is made to admit him to the psychiatric unit, to which he agrees. What would be the most appropriate medication to prescribe initially?
   A. Clozapine
   B. Lithium
   C. Quetiapine
   D. Alprazolam
   E. Chlordiazepoxide
   F. Fluoxetine

2. A 22-year-old male was brought in by his boss for "strange behavior." The patient sits in a chair and keeps repeating "waaawoo" to himself as he stares at the floor. His boss tells you that the man is a family friend

who recently emigrated from Namibia, and he does not think the man has any medical problems. Additionally, the patient's boss says that the patient started acting strangely 2 weeks ago, when his performance at work declined, and he said he kept hearing voices that no one else heard. On exam, his vital signs are normal, his pupils are 4 mm and equally reactive, he does not have nystagmus, he has moist mucus membranes, and there are no tremors observed. He is alert, oriented, and has intact memory. He has a clean UDS. What is your initial diagnosis?

A. Substance-induced psychosis
B. Schizophrenia
C. Schizoid personality disorder
D. Bipolar I
E. Brief psychotic disorder

3. A 24-year-old male graduate student comes to your office with complaints of chest tenderness and increased breast tissue. Last year his mother brought him to another psychiatrist, because he had been very anxious for 8 months that the government was watching him, and that the newspaper headlines carried special messages for him each day. They prescribed him a medication that he has been taking every day. Over the last few weeks, he has felt that his chest is growing and feeling sore. What medication was he likely taking?

A. Risperidone
B. Haloperidol decanoate
C. Escitalopram
D. Lamotrigine
E. Nortriptyline

Notes

ANSWERS: What Would Gunner Jess/Jim Do?

1. WWGJD? A 28-year-old man is brought to the hospital by police after he was found wandering on the railroad tracks. He appears malnourished and unkempt. Although he agrees to be interviewed, he often loses focus and will often stare at the wall for a few seconds and then laugh. He has no known medical history, but per a contacted family member he was hospitalized in a psychiatric institution when he was 19 for similar symptoms. He doesn't remember any of the meds he has ever taken. A urine toxicology screen and blood alcohol level are negative. A decision is made to admit him to the psychiatric unit, to which he agrees. What would be the most appropriate medication to prescribe initially?

Answer: C, Quetiapine

Explanation: This patient likely has schizophrenia given his internal preoccupation during the interview, his malnourished and unkempt appearance, and his history of institutionalization over 9 years ago (i.e., >6 months of these symptoms). Since we don't know if he failed antipsychotics before, an atypical antipsychotic such as quetiapine would be most appropriate. Other atypical antipsychotics, such as aripiprazole, risperidone, etc., also would be acceptable.

A. Clozapine → Incorrect. Clozapine is the most effective antipsychotic and would be effective in the treatment of this patient; however, the side effects associated with clozapine (agranulocytosis) are so severe that it is not used until multiple other antipsychotics have been tried and failed. Since we do not know if the patient failed medication in the past or if he simply has been non-compliant, it would not be appropriate to start him with clozapine.

B. Lithium → Incorrect. Lithium is the most effective treatment for bipolar affective disorder, but this patient does not display signs of mania. Buzz words for a manic psychosis include being found naked, racing thoughts, pacing the room, and delusions of grandeur. This patient is likely experiencing audiovisual hallucinations due to untreated schizophrenia.

D and E. Alprazolam and chlordiazepoxide → Incorrect. While benzodiazepines, such as alprazolam and chlordiazepoxide, can be helpful in the treatment of severe psychotic episodes, they are not the first-line treatment for a chronic psychotic disease, such as schizophrenia. In addition they would be used in conjunction with an antipsychotic medication.

F. Fluoxetine → Incorrect. Fluoxetine is an SSRI. There is no indication that this patient has any mood symptoms or history of mood disorders suggestive of schizoaffective disorder. SSRIs are not effective in the treatment of schizophrenia.

2. WWGJD? A 22-year-old male was brought in by his boss for "strange behavior." The patient sits in a chair and keeps repeating "waaawoo" to himself as he stares at the floor. His boss tells you that the man is a family friend who recently emigrated from the Namibia, and he does not think the man has any medical problems. Additionally, the patient's boss says that the patient **started acting strange 2 weeks ago**, when his performance at work declined and he said that he kept hearing voices that no one else heard. On exam, his vital signs are normal, his pupils are 4 mm and equally reactive, he does not have nystagmus, he has moist mucus membranes, and there are no tremors observed. He is alert, oriented, and has intact memory. He has a clean UDS. What is the most likely diagnosis?

Answer: E, Brief psychotic disorder

Explanation: This patient has been experiencing psychotic symptoms for less than a month. His recent immigration is likely the stressful impetus for his psychotic break. His physical exam is normal, and his mental status exam is strongly indicative of psychosis. People with psychosis can often have intact memory, orientation, and understanding of similarities or proverbs.

A. Substance-induced psychosis → Incorrect. PCP, cocaine, and LSD could all cause the patient's symptoms and be contributing to his decline at work. However, since he continues to experience the symptoms in the office despite having no physical exam findings of intoxication and having a negative urine drug screen, it is much less likely.

B. Schizophrenia → Incorrect. This patient presents with signs and symptoms of schizophrenia, but for diagnosis must have at least some symptoms for over 6 months. There is a 20%–50% chance that he will progress to develop schizophrenia, but initially the more accurate diagnosis is brief psychotic disorder.

C. Schizoid personality disorder → Incorrect. There are no indications that this patient has been having these symptoms for a long time or that he is socially withdrawn and isolated. Additionally, his overt psychotic symptoms are not consistent with schizoid personality disorder.

D. Bipolar I → Incorrect. While hallucinations and delusions are often the hallmark of Bipolar I, this patient does not show other signs of mania, such as distractibility, insomnia, grandiosity, or flight of ideas. Additionally, this patient's internal pre-occupation is less consistent with mania, which often presents with delusions of grandeur.

3. WWGJD? A 24-year-old male graduate student comes to your office with complaints of chest tenderness and increased breast tissue. Last year his mother brought him to another psychiatrist, because he had been very anxious for 8 months that the government was watching him, and that the newspaper headlines carried special messages for him each day. They prescribed him a medication that he has been taking every day. Over the last few weeks, he has felt that his chest is growing and feeling sore. What medication was he likely taking?

Answer: A, Risperidone.

Explanation: Given his history, it is very likely that this young man has schizophrenia. An effective first-line anti-psychotic is risperidone. A relatively common side effect of risperidone is gynecomastia and galactorrhea, which can present similarly to this.

B. Haloperidol decanoate → Incorrect. While haloperidol is a fine initial treatment for schizophrenia, the decanoate or depot form is often reserved for patients who have compliance issues. Additionally, the depot form is only prescribed after a trial run of the drug to prove that it is safe, and to determine the dose. Given that the patient says he is taking a medication every day, it is unlikely that he received haloperidol decanoate. Common side effects of haloperidol are akathisia (restlessness), nausea, vomiting, and dry mouth.

C. Escitalopram → Incorrect. Escitalopram is an SSRI that would not be indicated in this patient who has schizophrenia and likely received an antipsychotic. Additionally, SSRIs are not known to cause gynecomastia. Common SSRI side effects can include insomnia, restlessness, or insomnia, gastrointestinal (GI) upset or weight gain, and decreased libido.

D. Lamotrigine → Incorrect. Lamotrigine is a medication often used in the treatment of bipolar disorder. This patient's history is much more suggestive of schizophrenia rather than a mood disorder with psychotic features. Additionally, lamotrigine is not known to cause gynecomastia. A rare, but fatal side effect of lamotrigine is the dermatological condition Steven-Johnson syndrome.

E. Nortriptyline → Incorrect. Nortriptyline is a tricyclic antidepressant (TCA). TCAs are not used to treat schizophrenia. Nortriptyline is used to treat major depression, childhood nocturnal enuresis, and neuropathic pain. Its side effects include anticholinergic symptoms, such as dry eyes and constipation, but do not include gynecomastia.

Mood Disorders

Benjamin Yu, Hao-Hua Wu, Leo Wang, and Olga Achildi

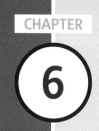

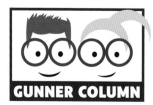

GUNNER COLUMN

Introduction

Mood disorders, at their core, mean some dysregulation of how we feel emotion on a day-to-day basis. There are normal responses to success, joy, adversity, stress, and catastrophe, and the human experience is the natural rhythm of these (and so many other!) emotions. However, when someone is persistently "up" or "down" with accompanying behaviors that may be causing damage to self or others, serious dysfunction and cascading consequences can have far-reaching effects. As with other diagnoses and therapeutic interventions in psychiatry and in medicine at large, the biggest question in evaluating a patient with mood disorders is how much the condition impairs the patient's function, relationships, and life.

The psychiatry shelf exam tends to emphasize the diagnosis of mood disorders over mechanism or management. This is partly due to the fact that our understanding of the mechanisms of psychiatric disease in general is still minimal at best. In short, we don't really know why and how a lot of these disorders arise. However, the emphasis on diagnosis means that you should work hard to commit diagnostic criteria (and/or helpful mnemonics!) to memory for this exam. Some of the trickiest diagnostic questions will require you to integrate your understanding of mood disorders, psychotic disorders, substance use disorders, and developmental disorders.

This chapter is divided into (1) unipolar disorders (one way), (2) bipolar disorders (two ways), and (3) unipolar or bipolar disorders (could be any which way). This organizing principle, applied to each question you see related to mood disorders, will help you narrow your differential and keep the many variants and subtypes of major disorders crystal clear in your mind.

Unipolar Disorders

A. Major Depressive Disorder (MDD) (>2 Weeks)

Buzz Words: SIGECAPS: anhedonia (loss of interest in activities one usually enjoys) + depressed or "down" mood + suicidal ideation + sleep troubles + trouble concentrating + psychomotor retardation (moving slower than usual) + low energy + lack of appetite + ≥2 weeks

Clinical Presentation: This is the most high-yield disease of this chapter. MDD can occur at any age with a chief complaint of one of the SIGECAPS symptoms, such as difficulty concentrating, in the setting of dysfunction at work or home. The most specific symptom of MDD on the shelf is anhedonia. Be on the lookout for the timing of symptoms (has to meet five out of nine SIGECAPS symptoms for at least 2 weeks) as well as any concomitant symptoms. If patient also has psychotic symptoms, MDD with psychotic features and schizoaffective disorder is also on the differential.

PPx: None

MoD: Unknown, but decreased serotonin in cerebrospinal fluid and possibly decreased norepinephrine and dopamine

Dx:
1. Urine drug screen (UDS) to r/o (rule out) substance use
2. Clinical diagnosis, satisfying 5/9 SIGECAPS criteria for greater than 2 weeks continuously (see criteria)

Tx/Mgmt:
1. **Selective serotonin reuptake inhibitors (SSRIs)** (Table 6.1) are generally considered first-line pharmacotherapy and are given a relatively safe side effect profile (effective trial considered to be medium-high dose for 6–8 weeks). Other reasonable first-line agents with differing side effect profiles: bupropion, mirtazapine, serotonin–norepinephrine reuptake inhibitors (SNRIs).
2. Tricyclic antidepressants (TCAs) and monoamine oxidase inhibitors (MAOIs) are older antidepressive agents with more side effects than SSRIs, but can be

QUICK TIPS

Psych disorders cannot be diagnosed in the setting of substance use. Thus, if patients exhibit symptoms of a mood disorder, always make sure their urine tox or drug screen is negative first. This is a high-yield point for both the shelf and clinics

99 AR

SIGECAPS

QUICK TIPS

Contraindications for antidepressive meds: (1) Bupropion/Wellbutrin → seizure disorder, (2) SNRIs → elevated blood pressure, and (3) TCAs → patients who do not tolerate anticholinergic side effects (e.g., elderly patients, or those who are fall risks)

TABLE 6.1 Common Selective Serotonin Reuptake Inhibitors

Brand Name	Trade Name
Fluoxetine	Prozac
Sertraline	Zoloft
Citalopram	Celexa
Escitalopram	Lexapro
Paroxetine	Paxil
Fluvoxamine	Luvox

Be familiar with both brand name and trade name. The trade name is useful for clinics only! Trade names for SSRIs are not tested on the shelf.

used in patients who cannot tolerate or do not respond to first line medications.

3. Electroconvulsive therapy (ECT) can be considered for patients with MDD unresponsive to medications and therapy.

4. Various forms of therapy (supportive, cognitive behavioral therapy (CBT), interpersonal) can be used in conjunction with medication.

B. Major Depressive Disorder With Psychotic Features

Buzz Words: Anhedonia (loss of interest in activities one usually enjoys) + mood-congruent **psychotic symptoms** + depressed or "down" mood + suicidal ideation + sleep troubles + trouble concentrating + psychomotor retardation (moving slower than usual) + low energy + lack of appetite + ≥2 weeks

Clinical Presentation: Patients report feeling down or depressed, or any of the vague individual somatic symptoms above (e.g., trouble sleeping, low energy, trouble concentrating, weight loss, lack of appetite) **in addition to psychotic symptoms.** Depression symptoms exist without psychotic symptoms, but psychosis cannot exist without depressive symptomatology. If psychosis does exist without depressive symptomatology, then the patient has schizoaffective disorder.

PPx: None

MoD: Unknown

Dx:

1. UDS to r/o substance use

2. Clinical diagnosis, satisfying 5/9 SIGECAPS criteria for greater than 2 weeks, along with psychotic symptoms that **only occur during episodes of mood symptoms**

Tx/Mgmt:

1. Antidepressant agents as for MDD without psychosis (SSRIs, SNRIs, mirtazapine, bupropion, TCAs, MAOIs) in addition to a reasonable antipsychotic agent (typical or atypical antipsychotics). Notably, the first-line combination is an SSRI + atypical antipsychotic.

2. ECT is also a reasonable treatment for patients who are refractory to medical management.

C. Major Depressive Disorder, Postpartum (With or Without Psychosis)

Buzz Words: Female + MDD + shortly after childbirth + ≥2 weeks

Clinical Presentation: On the shelf, this disorder only affects postpartum females with depressive symptomatology. Patients with a history of depression are at increased risk.

PPx: For patients with prior history of depression, PPx with antidepressants (SSRIs) or continuation of therapy has some evidence for preventing episodes of postpartum major depressive disorder.

Screening is still controversial. Some professional society guidelines (e.g., American College of Obstetrics and Gynecology) recommend screening all postpartum patients **at least once** for postpartum depression. Clinically useful tools for screening include the Edinburgh Postnatal Depression Scale or the more general Patient Health Questionnaire. Suggested timeframe of screening is **four to eight weeks after delivery**. Note that a growing trend is for some pediatricians to also screen parents/caretakers for postpartum depression at newborn visits.

MoD: Unknown

Dx:

1. UDS to r/o substance use
2. Clinical history and exam. Same clinical presentation as non-postpartum major depressive disorder. However, features specific to this diagnosis include depressive symptoms, delusions, or psychotic features **focusing on the newborn**, or on the **patient's inability to care for the baby**.

Note that the period defined as "postpartum" is not well defined, and can be defined anytime from 1 to 12 months after delivery of the baby. For most test purposes, look for **1–6 months postpartum** as the critical period for postpartum depression. Also, note that the *Diagnostic and Statistical Manual of Mental Disorders,* fifth edition (DSM-V) does not use "postpartum depression" as a diagnosis, but instead labels depressive episodes within 4 weeks after childbirth as a subtype of major depressive disorder "with peripartum onset."

Tx/Mgmt:

1. Assess need for acute inpatient hospitalization (severe depression, suicidality, frank psychosis). Of note, specifically look for indications that the baby would not be safe at home with the patient. In such cases, **separation of patient and child** is the number one priority.
2. Pharmacologic treatment, similar to major depressive disorder (first line = SSRIs, which have no contraindications at this time in breastfeeding (see below).

FOR THE WARDS

Although postpartum MDD only affects females on the shelf, note that paternal postpartum depression is an increasingly more clinically recognized entity that requires further study

QUICK TIPS

Postpartum blues, a less severe and much more common form of postpartum depression, usually has onset after birth, peaks by 5 days postpartum, and disappears by 10 days postpartum. If patient presents with depressive sxs in this 5- to 10-day postpartum timeframe, and is not severely depressed or psychotic, usually the correct answer is to **reassure the patient and follow up in 1–2 weeks.**

3. Therapy, especially interpersonal and supportive therapy, can be beneficial as well.
4. If patient is experiencing psychotic symptoms, patient can be started on antipsychotic medications (e.g., typical or atypical antipsychotics).

D. Persistent Depressive Disorder (Dysthymia)

Buzz Words: Up to 4/9 SIGECAPS symptoms + ≥2 years + cannot meet threshold for MDD at any time + symptomatic ≥1 year + symptom free <2 months at any point in time

Clinical Presentation: Dysthymia presents on the shelf as a patient with persistent depressive symptomatology over the course of at least 2 years. However, during the course of 2 years, the patient will never have more than 4/9 of SIGECAPS symptomatology.

PPx: None

MoD: Unknown

Dx:

1. UDS to r/o substance use
2. Clinical diagnosis via history and/or clinical exam. Patients will have chronic (potentially relapsing/remitting) depressive symptoms, but will not meet clinical criteria for major depressive disorder. DSM-V criteria indicate that patients cannot meet criteria for major depressive disorder **at any time**. Patients must demonstrate depressive symptoms for **at least 2 years**. In addition, patients **must be symptomatic for at least half** of that 2-year (or greater) span, and they **must not be symptom-free for more than 2 months at a time**

Tx/Mgmt:

1. Individual or combination therapy with psychotherapy and/or medications, with medication choice similar to that for major depressive disorder

Bipolar Disorders

A. Bipolar I Disorder (1 Week of Mania)

Buzz Words: 3/7 DIGFAST (see link below) symptoms for mania, either past or present + >1 week of mania

Clinical Presentation: Bipolar I is the second most high-yield topic of this chapter because a variety of pathology can mimic a manic episode, defined as an episode lasting over 1 week in which patients exhibit at least 3 of the DIGFAST signs/symptoms. Typically, patients with bipolar I will have a chief complaint of not sleeping, thoughts of grandeur, aggressiveness, or suicidality/homicidality. These patients can sometimes be brought to the

---

99 AR

DSM-V Criteria for MDD and Persistent Depressive Disorder

QUICK TIPS

Note that this diagnosis combines DSM-IV diagnoses of dysthymic disorder and chronic unipolar major depression (major depressive disorder lasting more than 2 years) because they were similar groups diagnostically and prognostically

---

QUICK TIPS

Some patients who present with persistent depressive disorder eventually DO have an episode meeting criteria for major depressive disorder. If this is the case, these patients have **double depression** (think of these patients as having a baseline of dysthymia with periodic MDD exacerbations). This is useful for clinics but not tested on the shelf.

---

99 AR

DIGFAST: Distractibility + Impulsivity + Grandiosity + Flight of Ideas + Activity (increased) + **Sleep deficit** + Talkativeness

hospital by family or police involuntarily after disruptive or dangerous behavior. Patients with a manic episode in the setting of psychosis should be considered on the shelf to be schizoaffective until proven otherwise.

PPx: None

MoD: Unknown

Dx:

1. UDS to r/o substance use
2. Clinical diagnosis via history and/or clinical exam

Tx/Mgmt:

1. In the acute setting with a patient who is severely manic, medication is initiated with **combination therapy** using
   a. **Lithium**
   b. **Antipsychotics** (typical or atypical)
   c. Mood stabilizers (usually **carbamazepine** or valproic acid). Common combinations include lithium + an antipsychotic or a mood stabilizer + an antipsychotic. If patients cannot tolerate combination therapy or present with a mild-moderate episode of mania, they can be started on monotherapy with one of these agents. Of note, these medications are also generally continued for maintenance therapy even after remission of symptoms. Benzodiazepines also can be used in the acute setting for urgent sedation, but are not recommended for maintenance therapy.
2. For patients who are refractory to medical treatment for mania, **ECT** is also an effective therapeutic intervention that can reduce duration and frequency of mania episodes.
3. For patients who present with depressive symptoms but who are known to have bipolar I or bipolar II disorder, SSRIs are NOT first line due to the risk of "switching" (inducing mania in a patient by treating depression). Empirical data is still unclear, but evidence-based pharmacotherapy options for these patients include quetiapine and Symbyax (olanzapine-fluoxetine combination pill). Other agents used to treat mania or used for general maintenance (such as lithium or mood stabilizers) do not currently have reliable data to indicate efficacy for the treatment of acute depressive episodes.

B. Bipolar II Disorder

Buzz Words: 1–2/7 DIGFAST symptoms (hypomania) + >4 days + no psychosis

---

99 AR

Definitions of Symptoms of Bipolar Disorder

99 AR

Changes in Bipolar Disorder Criteria from DSM-IV to DSM-V. **Useful for clinics but not for the shelf.**

QUICK TIPS

Patients can present with subtypes of bipolar I disorder; for example, a mixed episode (concurrent sxs of both mania and depression), or else can rapidly cycle between states of mania and depression "rapid cyclers."

Clinical Presentation: Patients with bipolar II disorder on the shelf have manic-like symptoms but do not reach the threshold of 3/7 DIGFAST symptomatology.

PPx: None

MoD: Unknown

Dx:

1. UDS to r/o substance use
2. Clinical diagnosis via history and/or clinical exam. Notably, to be defined as hypomania, a patient must have had symptoms for **at least 4 days**, and must not be experiencing psychotic symptoms or have the need for acute hospitalization. If the patient is psychotic or requires acute hospitalization, the patient is, by definition, experiencing a manic episode and is not eligible for the diagnosis of bipolar 2 disorder.

Tx/Mgmt:

1. Patients with bipolar II disorder are generally treated according to the same principles as patients with bipolar I disorder (see above).

Of note, hypomanic episodes are regarded as clinically less severe than manic episodes but not enough data exist to justify any differences in treatment at this time.

C. Cyclothymic Disorder

Buzz Words: <5/9 SIGECAPS + <3/7 DIGFAST + ≥2 years + does not meet criteria for bipolar disorder or MDD

Clinical Presentation: Look for patients with cyclic hypomanic and depressive symptoms who do not meet strict criteria for major depressive disorder or bipolar 2 disorder. Also follow the Rule of 2s: cycling between 2 states for 2 years with no normal state for >2 months in timeframe

PPx: None

MoD: Unknown

Dx:

1. UDS to r/o substance use
2. Clinical diagnosis via history and/or clinical exam. DSM-V criteria indicates that patients cannot meet criteria for bipolar I, bipolar 2, or major depressive disorder **at any time**. Patients must demonstrate alternating periods of hypomanic symptoms and depressive symptoms for at least 2 years. In addition, patients must be symptomatic for **at least half** of that 2 year (or greater) span, and they **must not be symptom-free for more than 2 months at a time.**

Tx/Mgmt:

1. Pharmacologic treatment for hypomanic or depressive symptoms is usually similar to treatment for bipolar I or

bipolar 2 disorder (e.g., appropriate pharmacotherapy for the acute presentation, along with considerations for maintenance and prevention of the "opposite" presentation).
2. Psychotherapy (supportive, interpersonal, CBT) is a reasonable intervention as well

D. Seasonal Affective Disorder (SAD)
Buzz Words: Manic/depressive symptomatology + occur during same season or time of year

Clinical Presentation: Patients with SAD present with mood symptoms (e.g., **manic** or **depressive** symptoms) that occur **cyclically** and **repeatedly** during the same season or same time of year (most commonly **winter**).

PPx: None

MoD: Unknown

Dx:
1. UDS to r/o substance use
2. Clinical diagnosis, with the key differentiating feature from MDD, bipolar I, or bipolar II disorder being the temporal association with a specific time of year or season

Tx/Mgmt:
1. For an acute episode with active symptoms, individual or combination therapy with
   a. light therapy
   b. appropriate medication management (**SSRIs** for depressive symptoms; atypical antipsychotics, lithium, or mood stabilizers for mania/hypomania)
   c. psychotherapy
2. Reasonable to consider maintenance therapy with any of the above, even when patient does not have active symptoms

Unipolar or Bipolar Disorders (or Can Be Associated With Such)

A. Suicidal Ideation/Attempt
Buzz Words: None

Clinical Presentation: The chief complaint of these patients is variable. They can present in acute medical distress to the emergency department (ED) or present less medically emergently in the outpatient setting. Often the chief complaint will just be "I feel suicidal."

Comorbid psychiatric conditions (schizophrenia, psychosis of any kind, substance use, depression, bipolar disorder) and past trauma correlate highly with suicidal ideation or attempts. Various social determinants of health—housing instability, intimate partner violence, traumatic living situation, food insecurity—can also contribute to suicide attempts. There are some classic associations that this test will often ask: the most important risk factor for a successfully completed suicide is **having a gun in the home**, and the most important risk factor for suicide attempts is **prior suicide attempts.**

PPx: None proven. The only two medications that have been shown in studies to decrease suicidality are **lithium and Clozaril**, but these medications are not generally given to patients who have suicidal ideation/ behavior unless they have another psychiatric indication for their use.

MoD: Unknown

Dx:

1. Clinical, from history or exam. Often seen in the context of other psychiatric symptoms (e.g., manic or depressive episode), substance use, or in the setting of the recent death of a loved one. Common methods seen in test questions: hanging, pill overdose, wrist-cutting

Tx/Mgmt:

1. Treat and stabilize the patient medically; for example, transfuse blood if actively bleeding, correct electrolyte abnormalities, administer appropriate antidotes (e.g., **NAC** for Tylenol OD, **naloxone** for opioid OD).
2. Evaluate acute need for inpatient hospitalization (medications, group and individual therapy, therapeutic environment).
3. Once suicidal ideation resolves, you can set up a close outpatient follow-up with a psychiatrist and/or therapist.

B. Substance-Induced Mood Disorder (Illegal or Prescribed)

Buzz Words: Use of substances + manic or depressive symptoms shortly thereafter

Clinical Presentation: Patients with substance-induced mood disorder will present in similar ways as patients with primary mood disorders—could be in acute manic episode, major depressive episode, suicidal ideation/ attempt. Like many other psychiatric disorders, home and family instability, along with high-risk living situations and trauma, correlate with substance use and substance-induced mood disorder.

PPx: None

MoD: Unknown, but this is especially of concern for substance users who start in teenage or young adult years, given that current research shows there is likely a long-term effect of early substance use on cognitive function and likelihood of psychiatric comorbidities

Dx:

1. UDS to r/o substance use
2. clinical, from history or exam. Can be any valence of mood disorder (mania, depression) with concomitant substance use of any sort (cocaine, alcohol, heroin, prescription opioids, benzodiazepines, inhalants, bath salts, stimulants, hallucinogens, etc.)

Tx/Mgmt:

1. Correct acute intoxication medically (if necessary).
2. Assess the need for acute inpatient hospitalization (if suicidal, severely depressed, manic, or desiring detoxification).
3. Long-term, work to stop the patient's substance use with various methods (counseling, 12-step programs, medications, such as naltrexone, disulfiram, methadone, or Suboxone). If the patient's substance use lessens or stops, assess if the mood disorder resolves with sobriety.

> **QUICK TIPS**
> For questions in which you are presented with a patient with mood disorder sxs, maintain a high suspicion for substance-induced mood disorder **unless you have definite evidence that the patient is not using drugs** (e.g., UDS negative)

C. Premenstrual Syndrome (PMS)

Buzz Words: Cyclical + comes and goes at same time of month + episodic

Clinical Presentation: Patients with PMS are post-menarche, and pre-menopause, though most women present in their teens or early adulthood rather than later on in adulthood. Presents with regular or cyclical presentation of a wide range of **physical** and/or **affective** symptoms and can range from headaches or bloating to depressed mood or irritability. Usually begins 3–5 days before the start of menses, lasts through first 2–5 days of menses. Notably, the patient should have **functional impairment** in order to merit a diagnosis of PMS.

PPx: None

MoD: Thought to be related to hormonal changes (specifically, fluctuating estrogen and progestin levels) that take place in the luteal phase of menstruation. These changes likely influence the body's other neurotransmitter systems—serotonin has been implicated as an important regulatory neurotransmitter, further research into other contributing factors is needed.

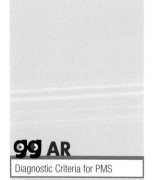

Dx:
1. Clinical history and exam

Tx/Mgmt:
 1. Menstrual diary for several months to confirm temporal relationship to menses.
 2. Nonpharmacologic interventions (meditation, relaxation techniques, sleep hygiene).
 3. Pharmacologic therapy—generally SSRIs (can be taken continuously or only during luteal phase of menstrual cycle) or oral contraceptive pills. Can also consider symptomatic management of somatic complaints (headaches, constipation, bloating, diarrhea, muscle aches).

D. Premenstrual Dysphoric Disorder (PMDD)
Buzz Words: Same as PMS

Clinical Presentation: Patients with PMDD present with cyclical somatic or affective complaint related temporally to patient's menstrual cycle. They can still have both physical and affective symptoms, but to fulfill this diagnosis the patient will tend to have **more severe mood/affect dysregulation.**

PPx: None

MoD: Same as PMS

Dx:
1. UDS to r/o substance use
2. Clinical history and exam

Tx/Mgmt:
1. Menstrual diary for several months to confirm temporal relationship to menses.
2. Assess whether patients meets criteria for acute inpatient hospitalization (acutely manic, depressed, psychotic, or suicidal).
3. Nonpharmacologic interventions (meditation, relaxation techniques, sleep hygiene).
4. Pharmacologic therapy—generally SSRIs (can be taken continuously or only during luteal phase of menstrual cycle) or oral contraceptive pills. Can also consider symptomatic management of somatic complaints (headaches, constipation, bloating, diarrhea, muscle aches).

E. Mood Disorder Secondary to Medical Condition
Buzz Words: Acute onset of disease or recent new medication + depression symptomatology + ≥2 weeks

Clinical Presentation: Pay attention to any medical history or medication lists provided in question stem! Patients may present similarly to any primary mood disorder (e.g., depression, suicidality, or bipolar disorder), but may be temporally related to the diagnosis or onset of a medical condition.

PPx: None

MoD: Variable

Dx:

1. Clinical history and exam. See Table 6.2.

Tx/Mgmt:

1. Consider whether primary mood disorder is reasonable or possible (temporally? symptomatically? Does this patient have a hx of psychiatric illness? Do the current symptoms match previous episodes of these psychiatric illnesses?).
2. Diagnose and treat underlying medical condition, then evaluate whether the mood disorder resolves or improves.

QUICK TIPS
Remember, patients with **any** medical condition may develop depressive/mood symptoms in reaction to diagnosis, setbacks, bad prognostic news, or hospitalization. On this exam, your task will often be to determine whether patients with comorbid medical conditions meet criteria for primary psychiatric diagnoses (e.g., MDD).

TABLE 6.2 Some Medical Causes of Mood Disorders

Neurologic	CVA, space-occupying lesion, Parkinson's, Huntington's, any variant of dementia, seizure disorder, delirium, multiple sclerosis
Metabolic	Diabetes, Cushing's, Addison's, hypoglycemia, hyper/hypothyroidism, hyper/hypocalcemia, vitamin/mineral deficiencies or excess (e.g., B12, thiamine), other electrolyte abnormalities
Rheumatologic	Lupus, rheumatoid arthritis
Medications	Corticosteroids, antimalarials, selective serotonin reuptake inhibitors (if used to treat patients who have bipolar disorders) amantadine, many more
Malignancy	Any cancer (lymphoma, pancreatic carcinoma tend to be emphasized on shelf exams)

Good to know for clinics but not needed for the shelf.

GUNNER PRACTICE

1. A 62-year-old man with a past medical history of longstanding type II diabetes mellitus, hypertension, and L-sided carotid occlusion presents to your outpatient clinic and says his mood has been "low" for the past 8 weeks. In addition, his wife has told him he has "been moving slower" recently, and his appetite, sleep, concentration, and energy have also been poor recently. He cannot think of a reason he feels this way. He denies suicidal ideation or suicide attempts. On review of systems, he states that the voices he has heard in his head "for a long time" are still present, though they may have increased in frequency in the last 2 weeks. Physical exam is significant for general dishevelment, loss of sensation to pinprick and light touch in a "stocking-and-glove" distribution, as well as a III/VI systolic ejection murmur heard most clearly at the upper left sternal border and an L carotid bruit. The remainder of the patient's neurological exam is intact. UDS is negative. What is the single most likely diagnosis in this patient that explains his recent mood symptoms?
   A. Mood disorder 2/2 general medical condition
   B. Substance-induced mood disorder
   C. Diabetic neuropathy
   D. Schizoaffective disorder
   E. Major depressive disorder with psychotic features

2. A 24-year-old male-to-female transgender patient comes to your office for a refill of medications. Her preferred name is "Willow," and her preferred pronouns are "she/her." She has been on hormone therapy for 3 years, but has not had any sexual reassignment surgeries. Her past medical history is otherwise significant for bipolar I disorder, oppositional defiant disorder, intermittent explosive disorder, asthma, eczema, and childhood obesity. Her current medications include lithium, combined hormone pills, aripiprazole, hydrocortisone cream, clonazepam, valproic acid, and albuterol PRN. The patient discloses that she has been the victim of cyberbullying, and that she has had suicidal thoughts recently. However, she is not currently suicidal and has not made a suicide plan. She otherwise denies all other depressive symptoms. Which of the following is most protective against this patient completing a suicide attempt in the future?
   A. Aripiprazole
   B. Clonazepam

   C. Lithium

   D. Inpatient hospitalization for suicidal ideation

   E. Valproic acid

3. A 42-year-old woman with a past medical history of epilepsy presents to the outpatient clinic and states she is feeling depressed. Her closest friend passed away unexpectedly 6 weeks ago, and she states she is having trouble adjusting. She says she feels hopeless about her future now that "my only friend is gone." She has lost interest in her hobbies, including painting and reading. She has lost 10 lbs in the last month and says she has no appetite. Additionally, she has no energy and says she spends all day lying on the couch and "staring at nothing." She denies suicidal thoughts or plan. Looking back in her medical chart, about 3 years ago the patient presented to the ED after a weeklong episode during which she spent $3000 on friendship bracelet materials, had unprotected sex with six partners in 3 days, and stayed up for 5 straight nights because she didn't need sleep. Currently, the patient is not taking any medications. At this time, what is a reasonable medication to start for this patient to treat her current symptoms?

   A. Haloperidol decanoate

   B. Bupropion

   C. Venlafaxine

   D. Fluoxetine

   E. Quetiapine

ANSWERS: What Would Gunner Jess/Jim Do?

1. WWGJD? A 62-year-old man with past medical history of longstanding type II diabetes mellitus, hypertension, and L-sided carotid occlusion presents to your outpatient clinic and says his mood has been "low" for the past 8 weeks. In addition, his wife has told him he has "been moving slower" recently, and his appetite, sleep, concentration, and energy have also been poor recently. He cannot think of a reason he feels this way. He denies suicidal ideation or suicide attempts. On review of systems, he states that the voices he has heard in his head "for a long time" are still present, though they may have increased in frequency in the last 2 weeks. Physical exam is significant for general dishevelment, loss of sensation to pinprick and light touch in a "stocking-and-glove" distribution, as well as a III/VI systolic ejection murmur heard most clearly at the upper left sternal border and a L carotid bruit. The remainder of the patient's neurological exam is intact. UDS is negative. What is the single most likely diagnosis in this patient that explains his recent mood symptoms?

Answer: D, Schizoaffective disorder

Explanation: The patient has an acute episode of mood symptoms, and he endorses multiple SIGECAPS symptoms. However, he also endorses a baseline of psychotic symptoms (e.g., voices in his head) that has a much longer time course than that of his mood symptoms. Importantly, he now has concurrent mood and psychosis symptoms, but has had psychosis symptoms without mood symptoms in the past.

A. Mood disorder 2/2 general medical condition → Incorrect. There is no likely relationship between the patient's medical conditions and his current symptoms. L carotid stenosis raises suspicion for CVA, but time course and clinical presentation of symptoms do not square with a CVA. In addition, the patient does not have any localizing symptoms that would raise concern for neurological events, such as CVA.

B. Substance-induced mood disorder → Incorrect. New-onset mood symptoms raise concern for substance use, but there are no other indications that the patient is taking substances, and his UDS is negative.

C. Diabetic neuropathy → Incorrect. While the patient does have likely diabetic neuropathy per his physical exam, this is a peripheral neuropathy that would not explain psychiatric symptoms.

   E. Major depressive disorder with psychotic features → Incorrect. For this diagnosis to be more strongly considered, this patient would have to endorse psychosis symptoms that only occur at the same time as his mood symptoms.

2. WWGJD? A 24-year-old male-to-female transgender patient comes to your office for a refill of medications. Her preferred name is "Willow", and her preferred pronouns are "she/her." She has been on hormone therapy for three years, but has not had any sexual reassignment surgeries. Her past medical history is otherwise significant for bipolar I disorder, oppositional defiant disorder, intermittent explosive disorder, asthma, eczema, and childhood obesity. Her current medications include lithium, combined hormone pills, aripiprazole, hydrocortisone cream, clonazepam, valproic acid, and albuterol PRN. The patient discloses that she has been the victim of cyberbullying, and that she has had suicidal thoughts recently. However, she is not currently suicidal and has not made a suicide plan. She otherwise denies all other depressive symptoms. Which of the following is most protective against this patient completing a suicide attempt in the future?

Answer: C, Lithium

   Explanation: The only two medications that have evidence in the literature supporting the fact that they are protective against future suicide risk are lithium and clozapine.

   A. Aripiprazole → Incorrect. This medication is an atypical antipsychotic that has not been shown to decrease future suicide risk. Clozapine is in the same class of medication and has been shown to decrease future suicide risk.

   B. Clonazepam → Incorrect. This medication is a benzodiazepine, which has not been shown to decrease future suicide risk.

   D. Inpatient hospitalization for suicidal ideation → Incorrect. This patient does not seem to be clinically depressed or suicidal and does not warrant immediate hospitalization. Additionally, being hospitalized has not been shown to decrease the future risk of suicide.

   E. Valproic acid → Incorrect. This medication is an antiepileptic/mood stabilizer, which has not been shown to decrease future suicide risk.

3. WWGJD? A 42-year-old woman with past medical history of epilepsy presents to outpatient clinic and states she is feeling depressed. Her closest friend passed away unexpectedly six weeks ago, and she states she is having trouble adjusting. She says she feels hopeless about her future now that "my only friend is gone." She has lost interest in her hobbies, including painting and reading. She has lost 10 lbs in the last month and says she has no appetite. Additionally, she has no energy and says she spends all day lying on the couch and "staring at nothing." She denies suicidal thoughts or plan. Looking back in her medical chart, about three years ago the patient presented to the ED after a week-long episode during which she spent $3000 on friendship bracelet materials, had unprotected sex with six partners in three days, and stayed up for five straight nights because she didn't need sleep. The patient currently is not taking any medications. At this time, what is a reasonable medication to start for this patient to treat her current symptoms?

Answer: E, Quetiapine

Explanation: Note that in this question, all the information provided is arguably important in guiding you to the correct answer (hence minimal strikethrough). This patient is presenting with symptoms meeting criteria for major depressive disorder, but also has a history of what sounds like a manic episode. Thus, in this situation, most reasonable first-line treatments for unipolar major depression are not efficacious. Additionally, treating bipolar depression with SSRIs has a small (~3% chance) of inducing mania, which is not a desirable outcome, obviously. Evidence-based treatment options for acute bipolar depression include quetiapine and Symbyax (fluoxetine/olanzapine combination pill).

A. Haloperidol decanoate → Incorrect. Typical antipsychotics are not the best medication to use for bipolar depression. Additionally, the decanoate form is a long-acting, injectable form of this medication that is used mostly in noncompliant patients who do not follow-up regularly. There are no clues given that this patient is noncompliant.

B. Buproprion → Incorrect. This medication can reasonably be used as a first-line medication for unipolar depression, but has no indication for bipolar depression. In addition, one of bupropion's major side effects is that it lowers the seizure threshold, and thus would not be the appropriate choice in a patient with a seizure disorder.

C. Venlafaxine → Incorrect. This medication, also a potential first-line medication for unipolar depression, has no indication for bipolar depression.

D. Fluoxetine → Incorrect. SSRIs, usually the first-line medication for unipolar depression, are not generally found to be efficacious for bipolar depression, and come with a small risk of "switching" or inducing mania (see above) in patients with bipolar depression.

Anxiety Disorders

*Thomas Knightly, Hao-Hua Wu, Leo Wang,
and Olga Achildi*

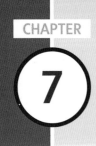

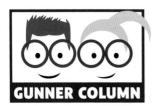

GUNNER COLUMN

Everyone experiences anxiety. We have all, at one time or another, questioned whether the anxiety we were feeling was normal or pathologic. That difference is central to this chapter. What makes anxiety pathologic is when it "causes significant distress or impairment in social, occupational, or other important areas of functioning." In fact, this notion runs central to all psychiatric disorders. That statement is found in the diagnostic criteria of nearly every psychiatric diagnosis.

There are several points to keep in mind while studying this chapter—the first being that for the purposes of learning, the diagnostic criteria have been simplified to include only the salient points. Keep a keen eye on the timing for each disease. Certain disorders, such as generalized anxiety disorder (GAD), cannot be diagnosed unless symptoms have been present for a certain amount of time (e.g., 6 months for GAD).

Next, each anxiety disorder is diagnosed only when the symptoms are not attributable to a substance/medication or to another medical condition. Keep this in mind when presented with a case where a substance or medical condition could be responsible for the symptoms of anxiety.

As you may realize, the mechanisms of the following diseases are multifactorial and not completely understood. As such, they are seldom tested. When tested, shelf questions typically are looking for an association with a particular area of the brain. If this is known for a disorder, it will be listed under its mechanism of disease.

Finally, there is considerable overlap between many of the anxiety disorders. Shelf examiners take advantage of this. Many questions will present a case with symptoms that are seen in more than one disorder. You must know what differentiates one disorder from another. Pay particular attention to what makes each disorder unique.

Panic Attack

Panic attack is not a mental disorder. Panic attacks may occur in the context of **any anxiety disorder**, as well as **other mental disorders** (e.g., major depressive disorder

[MDD], substance use disorders) or **medical conditions** (e.g., hyperthyroidism, asthma, pheochromocytoma). Panic attacks should be seen as a constellation of symptoms that occur within the context of any anxiety disorder but not specific to one. Panic attacks are characterized by an **abrupt surge of intense fear** that reaches a **peak within minutes**, during which time **four or more** of the following symptoms occur: (1) palpitations, (2) sweating, (3) trembling, (4) SOB, (5) feelings of choking, (6) chest pain/discomfort, (7) nausea or abdominal distress, (8) feeling dizzy/lightheaded, (9) chills or heat sensations, (10) paresthesias, (11) derealization or depersonalizations, (12) fear of losing control/going "crazy," and (13) fear of dying. Panic attacks are rarely tested directly on the shelf exam, but can show up as an answer choice, so be sure to know how to rule them out.

Generalized Anxiety and Related Disorders

A. Generalized Anxiety Disorder

Buzz Words: Fatigue + restlessness + irritability + inability to concentrate + muscle tension + sleep disturbances + lifelong + worse during times of stress + **≥6 months of symptoms**

Clinical Presentation: GAD is characterized by excessive worry and anxiety in **multiple** settings (e.g., work, school, family, finances, health, relationships) and at least **three of the following six symptoms**: (1) fatigue, (2) restlessness/feeling on edge, (3) irritability, (4) inability to concentrate/mind going blank, (5) muscle tension, and (6) sleep disturbances for a **minimum of 6 months**. Patients usually report **lifelong symptoms**, which are exacerbated in times of stress. What differentiates GAD from other anxiety disorders (e.g., social anxiety disorder, specific phobia) is that it occurs in more than one setting. For example, a patient with GAD may present with symptoms of a specific phobia, but he/she will also have symptoms of anxiety in another setting (e.g., worry about finances, school grades).

PPx: None

MoD: Multifactorial, unimportant for shelf exam

Dx:

1. Urine drug screen (UDS) to r/o (rule out) concomitant drug use. Psych disorders cannot be diagnosed in the setting of substance use.

> **MNEMONIC**
> GAD Symptoms: C-FIRMS
> **C**oncentration
> **F**atigue
> **I**rritability
> **R**estlessness
> **M**uscle tension
> **S**leep disturbances

2. Excessive worry in multiple settings (e.g., work, school, family, finances, health, relationships).
3. At least three of the following six symptoms:
   (i) Fatigue
   (ii) Restlessness/feeling on edge
   (iii) Irritability
   (iv) Inability to concentrate/mind going blank
   (v) Muscle tension
   (vi) Sleep disturbances
4. For a minimum of 6 months.

Tx/Mgmt:

1. First-line treatment includes cognitive behavioral therapy (CBT) ± pharmacotherapy.
2. First-line pharmacotherapy includes selective serotonin reuptake inhibitor/serotonin–norepinephrine reuptake inhibitor (SSRI/SNRI), buspirone (serotonin 5-HT$_{1A}$ receptor agonist), or benzos.

Buspirone (BuSpar) and SSRI/SNRIs take 2–3 weeks before effects are evident.

Benzos may be used during this interim; however, their use should be limited due to their potential for dependency.

Most commonly, CBT + SSRI/SNRI is the treatment of choice.

B. Panic Disorder

Buzz Words: Unexpected panic attacks + avoidance + worry about future panic attacks + decreased amygdala + ≥1 month

Clinical Presentation: Panic disorder is characterized by **multiple unexpected** panic attacks. Patients experience **persistent worry about having future panic attacks** and often modify their behavior to avoid having another attack (**avoidance**). What differentiates panic disorder from other anxiety disorders with panic attacks is the **unexpected nature (no known trigger)** of the attacks.

Panic attacks that occur in the context of any other anxiety disorder are expected (e.g., triggered by social situations in social anxiety disorder, by phobic objects or situations in specific phobia) and thus would not meet criteria for panic disorder. Panic attacks may also be caused by medical conditions (see "Anxiety Due to a Medical Condition") or substances (see "Substance Induced Anxiety") and therefore are not unexpected and do not meet criteria for panic disorder.

PPx: None

MoD: Unknown; however, is correlated with a **decreased volume of the amygdala**

MNEMONIC

Important Panic Disorder Points:
My **Amygdala Avoids Multiple Unexpected Future** attacks

Dx:
1. Recurrent, unexpected panic attacks.
2. At least one of the attacks has been followed by 1 month (or more) of one or both of the following:
   (i) Persistent concern or worry about additional panic attacks or their consequences (e.g., losing control, having a heart attack, "going crazy").
   (ii) A significant maladaptive change in behavior related to the attacks (e.g., behaviors designed to avoid having panic attacks, such as avoidance of exercise or unfamiliar situations).
3. Panic disorder is not diagnosed if the panic attacks are judged to be a direct physiological consequence of a substance or another medical condition.

Tx/Mgmt:
1. Immediate treatment—benzos.
2. Long-term treatment—SSRI/SNRI ± CBT. Benzos may be used during the 2–3 weeks period that it takes for SSRI/SNRIs to take effect; however, they should not be used long-term because of their dependency potential.

C. Agoraphobia

Buzz Words: Panic disorder + open spaces + public transport + large crowds + alone + no one nearby to help + avoidance

Clinical Presentation: Agoraphobia refers to a fear of places from which escape might be difficult. Most commonly, agoraphobia develops as a complication in patients with panic disorder. That is, **fear of having a panic attack in a place from which escape would be difficult** is the cause of the agoraphobia. As such, patients avoid these places or insist that they be accompanied by a friend or family member. When experiencing fear and anxiety cued by such situations, individuals typically experience thoughts that something terrible might happen. At its extreme, patients may refuse to leave their home entirely. Although agoraphobia almost always coexists with panic disorder, it is classified as a separate condition.

PPx: None

MoD: Multifactorial, unimportant for shelf exam

Dx:
1. Marked fear or anxiety about two or more of the following five situations:
   (i) Using public transportation (e.g., buses, trains, ships, planes)
   (ii) Being in open spaces (e.g., parking lots, bridges, marketplaces)

99 AR

Agoraphobia on "The Doctors"

   (iii) Being in enclosed spaces (e.g., shops, theaters, cinemas)
   (iv) Standing in line or being in a crowd
   (v) Being outside of the home alone
2. The individual fears or avoids these situations because of thoughts that escape might be difficult or help might not be available in the event of developing panic-like symptoms or other incapacitating or embarrassing symptoms (e.g., fear of falling in the elderly, fear of incontinence).
3. The agoraphobic situations are actively avoided, require the presence of a companion, or are endured with intense fear or anxiety.

Tx/Mgmt: Same as panic disorder:
1. Immediate treatment—benzos.
2. Long-term treatment—SSRI/SNRI ± CBT.

D. Hyperventilation Syndrome

Buzz Words: Rapid breathing + shallow breathing + light-headedness + carpopedal spasms + paresthesias + syncope

Clinical Presentation: Hyperventilation syndrome is characterized by **rapid and deep breathing** for several minutes by an individual who is often **unaware** he/she is doing so. This results in an excessive loss of CO_2, resulting in respiratory alkalosis. In addition, cerebral vasoconstriction results from low cerebral tissue PCO_2. Patients experience symptoms of light-headedness, dyspnea, paresthesias, chest pain, palpitations, carpopedal spasms, and diaphoresis. Finally, syncope may occur. It can present similarly to a panic attack. It can be differentiated from a panic attack by the resolution of symptoms with slow breathing techniques.

PPx: None

MoD: Unknown; however, it is believed to be solely psychological with no organic etiology

Dx:
1. There is no gold standard diagnostic test or criteria. Diagnosis is based upon clinical suspicion and absence of findings to support an alternative diagnosis.

Tx/Mgmt:
1. Immediate treatment—patient reassurance that the symptoms are due to rapid breathing and not a more serious cause, and slow breathing techniques that raise plasma PCO_2 and thus abort the symptoms. Forced rebreathing of CO_2 by breathing

into a paper bag is no longer recommended, as it can cause significant hypoxemia and consequent complications.

2. Long-term treatment—behavioral therapy focused upon breathing retraining.

E. Social Anxiety Disorder (Social Phobia)

Buzz Words: Scrutiny + embarrassment + performance + presentation

Clinical Presentation: Social anxiety disorder is characterized by **persistent anxiety about social situations** due to **fear of scrutiny and embarrassment**, resulting in avoidance, distress, and social-occupational dysfunction. Panic attacks are common and are exclusively in response to social interactions in which the patient fears negative evaluation by others. Must differentiate from panic disorder (i.e., unexpected panic attacks), GAD (i.e., anxiety in multiple setting, not just social situations), specific phobia (i.e., not diagnosed when the phobia is strictly to social situations), avoidant personality disorder (i.e., they have a broader avoidance pattern), and schizoid personality disorder (i.e., lack of desire for close relationships, emotionally detached, and exhibits a flat affect).

Performance-only type of social anxiety disorder— Individuals do not fear nonperformance social situations. Classically, the individual enjoys socializing with friends but is anxious about speaking in front of a group or performing on stage.

PPx: None

MoD: Multifactorial, unimportant for shelf exam

Dx:

1. Marked fear or anxiety about one or more social situations in which the individual is exposed to possible scrutiny by others.
2. The individual fears that he or she will act in a way or show anxiety symptoms that will be negatively evaluated (e.g., will be humiliating or embarrassing; will lead to rejection or offend others).
3. Social situations are avoided or endured with intense fear or anxiety.
4. For a minimum of 6 months.

Tx/Mgmt:

1. First-line treatment—SSRI/SNRI + CBT,
2. β-blockers for performance-only type. β-blockers helps control the autonomic response (i.e., tremors, tachycardia, diaphoresis).

gg AR

Exposure Therapy of a Bird Phobia

F. Specific Phobia

Buzz Words: Spiders + flying + needles + heights

Clinical Presentation: Specific phobia is characterized by a strong, exaggerated fear of a **specific object or situation** for **> 6 months.** Common types include flying, heights, animals, injections, blood, bridges, elevators. It must be differentiated from panic disorder (i.e., unexpected panic attacks), social anxiety disorder (i.e., panic due to social situations), and GAD (i.e., anxiety in multiple settings).

PPx: None

MoD: Multifactorial, unimportant for shelf exam

Dx:

1. Fear or anxiety about a specific object or situation.
2. The phobic object or situation almost always provokes immediate fear or anxiety.
3. The phobic object or situation is actively avoided or endured with intense fear or anxiety.
4. For a minimum of 6 months.

Tx/Mgmt:

1. First-line treatment—behavioral therapy, specifically using exposure techniques.
2. Benzos can be used acutely but should have a limited role and not be used long term due to potential for dependency.

MNEMONIC

Common medical causes:

HPA axis
Hyperthyroidism
Pheochromocytoma
Asthma

G. Anxiety Disorder Due to Another Medical Condition

BuzzWords: Asthma + hyperthyroidism + pheochromocytoma

Clinical Presentation: Anxiety disorder due to another medical condition is diagnosed when the panic attacks are a direct physiological consequence of another medical condition (e.g., hyperthyroidism, pheochromocytoma, asthma, COPD, arrhythmias, seizure disorder).

PPx: None

MoD: Varied based upon particular disease process

Dx:

1. Panic attacks or anxiety is predominant in the clinical picture.
2. There is evidence from the history, physical examination, or laboratory findings that the disturbance is the direct pathophysiological consequence of another medical condition.
3. The disturbance is not better explained by another mental disorder.
4. The disturbance does not occur exclusively during the course of a delirium.

Tx/Mgmt: Treatment of the underlying medical condition

H. Substance/Medication-Induced Anxiety Disorder

Buzz Words: Albuterol + levothyroxine + acute intoxication + withdrawal + overmedication

Clinical Presentation: Substance/medication-induced anxiety disorder is the direct result of a toxic substance. It can occur due to intoxication (e.g., cocaine, amphetamines, caffeine), withdrawal (e.g., alcohol, benzos), or after exposure to a medication (e.g., albuterol, levothyroxine)

PPx: None

MoD: Varied based upon particular substance

Dx:

1. Panic attacks or anxiety is predominant in the clinical picture.
2. The symptoms developed during or soon after substance intoxication or withdrawal or after exposure to a medication.
3. The involved substance/medication is capable of producing the symptoms that can cause panic attacks or anxiety.
4. The disturbance does not occur exclusively during the course of a delirium.

Tx/Mgmt: Removal of the offending substance or supportive treatment if withdrawal is the etiology of the anxiety.

Obsessive-Compulsive Disorder and Related Disorders

A. Obsessive-Compulsive Disorder (OCD)

Buzz Words: Contamination + hand washing + checking door locks + checking stove is off + praying repeatedly + counting + order + intrusive thoughts

Clinical Presentation: OCD is characterized by intrusive, anxiety-provoking, unwanted thoughts, urges, or images (obsessions) and attempts to suppress the obsessions with repeated behaviors or mental acts (compulsions). Common obsessions include worries about contamination, doubt (e.g., forgetting to lock the door or turn off the stove), and symmetry/order. Common compulsions include ritualistic hand washing, ordering, checking (e.g., door locked, oven off), praying, counting, and repeating words silently. The obsessions or compulsions are **time consuming** (i.e., takes more than 1 hour per day). **Individuals recognize the irrational nature of their behavior but feel unable to stop.** OCD must be differentiated from body dysmorphic disorder (i.e., obsessions and compulsions only focused on appearance),

99 AR

Interesting 20/20 Episode on Howie Mandel's struggle With OCD (relevant study break?)

trichotillomania (i.e., lack of obsessive thoughts and only one compulsive activity versus multiple in OCD), and obsessive-compulsive personality disorder (OCPD) (i.e., ego-syntonic vs. ego-dystonic). It also has a high comorbidity with Tourette syndrome.

PPx: None

MoD: Abnormalities in the orbitofrontal cortex and basal ganglia

Dx:

1. Presence of obsessions, compulsions, or both.
2. The obsessions and compulsions are time consuming (e.g., take more than 1 hour per day).

Tx/Mgmt:

1. First-line treatment—exposure and response prevention (i.e., a type of CBT) +/− an SSRI (especially fluvoxamine)
2. Clomipramine or antipsychotic augmentation for treatment nonresponse
3. Deep-brain stimulation for treatment of severe or refractory cases

MNEMONIC
OCD mechanism:
Orbitofrontal Cortex & Basal Ganglia

99 AR
Body Dysmorphic Disorder Full-Length Documentary (for enjoyment purposes only—will not get you points on your exam!)

B. Body Dysmorphic Disorder=

Buzz Words: Physical appearance + physical defect + perceived defect + feeling ugly

Clinical Presentation: Body dysmorphic disorder is characterized by **intense preoccupation** with a **perceived defect in physical appearance**. The defect is not observable or appears slight to others. In response to the preoccupation, individuals may perform repetitive behaviors such as excessive mirror checking/grooming or mental acts (e.g., comparing). It must be differentiated from OCD (i.e., obsessions and compulsions focused on more than just appearance), conversion disorder (i.e., preoccupation with a neurological symptom, not appearance), and somatic symptom disorder (i.e., preoccupation with a physical symptom, not appearance). Also, skin picking and hair pulling can be considered part of body dysmorphic disorder if the intention is to improve the perceived defect. However, if this is not the intention, then excoriation disorder and trichotillomania should be diagnosed respectively. Finally, in an individual with an eating disorder, preoccupation with weight and body image is considered a symptom of the eating disorder, and thus body dysmorphic disorder is not diagnosed.

PPx: None

MoD: Multifactorial, unimportant for shelf exam

Dx:
1. Preoccupation with one or more perceived defects or flaws in physical appearance that are not observable or appear slight to others.
2. At some point during the course of the disorder, the individual has performed repetitive behaviors (e.g., mirror checking, excessive grooming, skin picking, reassurance seeking) or mental acts (e.g., comparing his or her appearance with that of others) in response to the appearance concerns.
3. The preoccupation with appearance does not occur in an individual who meets diagnostic criteria for an eating disorder.

Tx/Mgmt:
1. First-line treatment—education about the illness and CBT ± SSRI/SNRI.

C. Hoarding Disorder
Buzz Words: Clutter + clustered living areas + unable to discard

Clinical Presentation: Hoarding disorder is characterized by **accumulation** of a large number of possessions that may cluster living areas to the point that they are unusable. Patients experience intense **distress when attempting to discard possessions**, regardless of their actual value. Social isolation due to embarrassment (i.e., not being able to invite people to their home) often occurs.

PPx: None

MoD: Multifactorial, unimportant for shelf exam

Dx:
1. Persistent difficulty discarding or parting with possessions, regardless of their actual value.
2. This difficulty is due to a perceived need to save the items and to distress associated with discarding them.
3. The difficulty discarding possessions results in the accumulation of possessions that congest and clutter active living areas and substantially compromises their intended use.

Tx/Mgmt:
1. First-line treatment—CBT.

D. Trichotillomania
Buzz Words: Bald spot + blading + hat wearing + hair loss

Clinical Presentation: Trichotillomania is characterized by **recurrent hair pulling** resulting in **hair loss**. The individual makes **repeated attempts to decrease/stop the**

hair pulling. The individual experiences psychological distress as a result of the hair pulling. It shares similarities with OCD in that there is increased tension prior to the hair pulling and a relief of tension or gratification after the hair pulling. However, it differs from OCD in that individuals with trichotillomania lack intrusive obsessive thoughts and only experience this one compulsive activity, while those with OCD experience multiple compulsions. It must also be differentiated from body dysmorphic disorder (i.e., diagnosed when the hair pulling is with the intent to improve the appearance of the perceived defect).

PPx: None

MoD: Multifactorial, unimportant for shelf exam

Dx:

1. Recurrent pulling out of one's hair, resulting in hair loss.
2. Repeated attempts to decrease or stop hair pulling.

Tx/Mgmt:

1. First-line treatment—habit reversal training (i.e., a form of CBT).

E. Excoriation Disorder

Buzz Words: Scratches + skin picking + multiple skin infections

Clinical Presentation: Excoriation disorder is characterized by recurrent skin picking with repeated **unsuccessful attempts to decrease or stop picking.** The most commonly picked sites are the face, arms, and hands. It is associated with high rates of comorbid OCD. However, it differs from OCD in that individuals with excoriation disorder lack intrusive, obsessive thoughts and only experience this one compulsive activity, while those with OCD experience multiple compulsions. It must also be differentiated from body dysmorphic disorder (i.e., diagnosed when the skin picking is done with the intent to improve the appearance of the perceived defect).

PPx: None

MoD: Multifactorial, unimportant for shelf exam

Dx:

1. Recurrent skin picking resulting in skin lesions.
2. Repeated attempts to decrease or stop skin picking.
3. The skin picking is not attributable to the physiological effects of a substance (e.g., cocaine) or another medical condition (e.g., scabies).

Tx/Mgmt:

1. First-line treatment—CBT + SSRI/SNRI

Trauma and Stress-Related Disorders

A. Posttraumatic Stress Disorder (PTSD)

Buzz Words: Veteran + combat exposure + rape victim + flashbacks + nightmares + amnesia + hypervigilance

PPx: None

MoD: Associated with **decreased hippocampal volume**

Dx:

1. UDS
2. H&P looking for
   (i) Exposure to actual or threatened death, serious injury, or sexual violence
   (ii) Intrusive symptoms (e.g., intrusive memories, dreams, flashbacks)
   (iii) Persistent avoidance of stimuli associated with the traumatic event (e.g., avoidance of external reminders that arouse distressing memories, thoughts, or feelings)
   (iv) Negative alterations in cognitions and mood (e.g., inability to remember an important aspect of the traumatic event, persistent and exaggerated negative beliefs, persistent negative emotional state, markedly diminished interest or participation in significant activities, feelings of detachment or estrangement from others, persistent inability to experience positive emotions),
   (v) Marked alterations in arousal and reactivity (e.g., irritable behavior, angry outbursts, self-destructive behavior, hypervigilance, sleep disturbance). High comorbidity with substance use disorder.
   (vi) Duration of the disturbance is more than 1 month.

Tx/Mgmt:

1. First-line treatment—trauma-focused CBT ± SSRI/SNRIs

99 AR

What PTSD Is Really Like

MNEMONIC

PTSD Mechanism:
   Poke the Stressed Hippo

B. Acute Stress Disorder

Buzz Words: Same as PTSD

Clinical Presentation: Acute stress disorder is characterized by the development of characteristic symptoms following exposure to a traumatic event. The traumatic event, characteristic symptoms, and diagnostic criteria are similar to those of PTSD, with the exceptions that **the symptoms develop within 1 month of the trauma** and that **the symptoms last a minimum of 3 days and a maximum of 1 month.** It must also be differentiated from adjustment disorder (i.e., lack of life-threatening trauma).

PPx: None

MoD: Multifactorial, unimportant for shelf exam
Dx: Similar criteria as PTSD with the following exceptions:
1. The symptoms begin within 1 month of the trauma.
2. The symptoms last more than 3 days but less than 1 month.

Tx/Mgmt: Same as PTSD

C. Adjustment Disorder

Buzz Words: Divorce + breakup + work stresses + anxiety symptoms + depressive symptoms + within 3 months of stressor

Clinical Presentation: Adjustment disorder is characterized by emotional or behavioral symptoms (e.g., anxiety, depression, disturbance of conduct) that develop within 3 months in response to an identifiable stressor and last no longer than 6 months after the stressor ends. The distress is in excess of what would be expected by exposure to the stressor. Common stressors include marital and work difficulties. Adjustment disorder is not diagnosed if the symptoms meet criteria for another disorder. For example, an individual may develop symptoms in response to a stressor; however, if the symptoms are enough to make a diagnosis of MDD or another anxiety disorder, then that diagnosis supersedes adjustment disorder and adjustment disorder is not diagnosed. Accordingly, if the depressive or anxiety symptoms are not enough to meet criteria for MDD or an anxiety disorder, then adjustment disorder with depressive symptoms or adjustment disorder with anxiety is diagnosed, respectively. Adjustment disorder can be differentiated from acute stress disorder and PTSD by its lack of a life-threatening trauma.

PPx: None
MoD: Multifactorial, unimportant for shelf exam
Dx:
1. The development of emotional or behavioral symptoms in response to an identifiable stressor occurring within 3 months of the onset of the stressor.
2. Marked distress that is out of proportion to the severity or intensity of the stressor.
3. The symptoms do not represent normal bereavement.
4. Once the stressor has terminated, the symptoms do not persist for more than an additional 6 months.

Tx/Mgmt:
1. First-line treatment—psychotherapy

GUNNER PRACTICE

1. A 19-year-old college freshman presents to her school's health center with complaints of difficulty concentrating while studying for her upcoming finals. She is concerned that she has ADHD and asks if Adderall will help her. Upon questioning, you learn that she has felt on edge, has been sleeping poorly, and has been more irritable than normal since the start of the college year, 10 months ago. She stresses about getting all A's but says she has always been this way. She rarely goes to parties with friends due to worries she will embarrass herself dancing. She often frets about her ability to repay her student loans after graduation and occasionally skips meals to save a few dollars. She admits she has always been a "penny pincher." She denies any substance use other than an occasional sip of wine on the weekends. What is the most likely diagnosis?
   A. Social anxiety disorder
   B. Adjustment disorder
   C. Generalized anxiety disorder
   D. Specific phobia

2. A 46-year-old woman who is known to you comes to the office for a check-up. She tells you that she was raped by a coworker after a company party on New Year's Eve. She says that she can no longer recall the details of the incident as she has "blocked it out." She states for the past 4 months she has not been able to get a good night's sleep and frequently wakes up to nightmares. While the perpetrator no longer works at her company, she now tries to work from home as much as possible because her work office is a reminder of what happened. She tells you that she sometimes blames herself for what happened, saying if only she hadn't worn such a tight dress then maybe she wouldn't have been a target. What is the most likely diagnosis?
   A. Adjustment disorder
   B. PTSD
   C. Acute stress disorder
   D. Dissociative amnesia
   E. B + D
   F. C + D

3. An 18-year-old male presents to your office at the insistence of his mother. The mother states that the boy is obsessed with his looks, to the point where he spends several hours per day in front of the mirror. The boy doesn't see anything wrong with this. He says that he hates the way his

"fat cheeks" look. He has scratches on both sides of his face from "trying to rip out the excess fat in my cheeks." He also compulsively picks at his facial hair, as it "makes my cheeks look even fatter." What is the most likely diagnosis?

A. Excoriation disorder

B. Trichotillomania

C. Body dysmorphic disorder

D. Obsessive-compulsive disorder

Notes

ANSWERS: What Would Gunner Jess/Jim Do?

1. **WWGJD?** A 19-year-old college freshman presents to her school's health center with complaints of **difficulty concentrating** while studying for her upcoming finals. She is concerned that she has ADHD and asks if Adderall will help her. Upon questioning, you learn that she has **felt on edge,** has been **sleeping poorly,** and has been more **irritable** than normal since the start of the college year, **10 months ago.** She **stresses about getting all A's** but says she has **always been this way.** She **rarely goes to parties** with friends due to **worries she will embarrass herself** dancing. She often **frets about** her ability to repay her student loans after graduation and occasionally **skips meals to save a few dollars.** She admits she has **always been a "penny pincher."** She **denies any substance use** other than an occasional sip of wine on the weekends. What is the most likely diagnosis?

   Answer: C, Generalized anxiety disorder

   Explanation: This individual has anxiety across multiple settings (e.g., school, social, financial) along with the following symptoms: feeling on edge, sleeping poorly, irritability, and difficulty concentrating. She has had these symptoms for greater than 6 months, thus making GAD the most likely diagnosis.

   A. Social anxiety disorder → Incorrect. While she does display symptoms of anxiety in social situations, she also displays symptoms of anxiety in other settings as well, thus making GAD the more appropriate diagnosis.

   B. Adjustment disorder → Incorrect. Her worries about grades and money predate her recent stressor of going to college. Thus this is less likely adjustment disorder and more likely GAD with worsening symptoms during a time of stress (i.e., college).

   D. Specific phobia → Incorrect. Her anxiety symptoms occur in multiple settings, thus making specific phobia (anxiety occurring in one particular setting/situation) incorrect.

2. **WWGJD?** A 46-year-old woman who is known to you comes to the office for a check-up. She tells you that she was **raped** by a coworker after a company party on New Year's Eve. She says that she can **no longer recall the details of the incident** as she has "blocked it out." She states for the past **4 months** she has **not been able to get a good night's sleep** and frequently wakes up to **nightmares.** While the perpetrator no longer works

at her company, she now tries to work from home as much as possible because her **work office is a reminder of what happened.** She tells you that she sometimes **blames herself** for what happened saying if only she hadn't worn such a tight dress then maybe she wouldn't have been a target. What is the most likely diagnosis?

Answer: B, PTSD

Explanation: This individual has experienced trauma of sexual violence. She has intrusive symptoms (i.e., nightmares), persistent avoidance of external reminders (i.e., her work), negative alterations in mood (i.e., inability to remember aspects of the event), alterations in arousal (i.e., sleep disturbances), and symptoms that have lasted longer than 1 month.

A. Adjustment disorder → Incorrect. With adjustment disorder, the inciting event is not life threatening, nor sexual assault.

C. Acute stress disorder → Incorrect. Acute stress disorder symptoms do not last longer than 1 month.

D. Dissociative amnesia → Incorrect. Dissociative amnesia is not diagnosed as a separate diagnosis when full criteria for PTSD is met.

E. B + D → Incorrect. Dissociative amnesia is not diagnosed as a separate diagnosis when full criteria for PTSD is meet.

F. C + D → Incorrect. Dissociative amnesia is not diagnosed as a separate diagnosis when full criteria for PTSD is meet.

3. **WWGJD?** An 18-year-old male presents to your office at the insistence of his mother. The mother states that the boy is **obsessed with his looks,** to the point where he spends **several hours per day** in front of the mirror. The boy doesn't see anything wrong with this. He says that he **hates** the way his **"fat cheeks"** look. He has **scratches** on both sides of his **face** from "trying to **rip out the excess fat in my cheeks."** He also compulsively **picks at his facial hair,** as it "makes my cheeks look even fatter." What is the most likely diagnosis?

Answer: C, Body dysmorphic disorder

Explanation: This individual has a preoccupation with a perceived defect in his physical appearance (i.e., his cheeks), has performed repetitive behaviors (mirror checking, skin picking, and hair pulling) in response to his appearance concerns, and his preoccupation is not in the setting of an eating disorder.

A. Excoriation disorder → Incorrect. Skin-picking can be part of body dysmorphic disorder when the picking is done to improve the appearance of the perceived defect. He is picking at his skin in for this reason; thus, excoriation disorder is not diagnosed.

B. Trichotillomania → Incorrect. Hair pulling can be part of body dysmorphic disorder when the pulling is done to improve the appearance of the perceived defect. He is pulling out his facial hair for this reason; thus trichotillomania is not diagnosed.

D. Obsessive-compulsive disorder → Incorrect. For a diagnosis of OCD to be made over body dysmorphic syndrome, this individual would need his obsessions and compulsions to be focused on more than just his appearance. This is not the case; thus, OCD is not diagnosed.

In response to the preoccupation, individuals may perform repetitive behaviors such as excessive mirror checking/grooming or mental acts (e.g., comparing). It must be differentiated from OCD (i.e., obsessions and compulsions focused on more than just appearance).

Somatoform Disorders

Leo Wang, Hao-Hua Wu, and Olga Achildi

Introduction

Somatoform disorders are some of the most unique diseases that psychiatrists face on a day-to-day basis. As a result, questions on somatoform disorders on the psychiatry shelf usually stand out in that they won't seem as obvious as others.

By definition, somatoform disorders mean that the patient experiences **symptoms** without any medical evidence for a disease or problem. Most of the time, somatoform disorders occur in the setting of other psychiatric comorbidities—most commonly, anxiety and depression. Classically, these are the diseases for which a therapist or psychiatrist might say, "It's all in your head." However, it's important to remember that these patients nonetheless still feel pain or other physical symptoms and should be treated as such. As a rule of thumb, these patients require more care than normal medical patients, and the way you approach these patients should be commensurate with that. Never, ever dismiss a patient, no matter how a question stem presents him/her, and always offer follow-up appointments if necessary. Always try to rule out nonpsychiatric causes for symptoms.

In general, the prophylaxis for most somatoform disorders will be to treat psychiatric comorbidities. The mechanism is poorly understood for all of these diseases, but generally all the somatoform disorders are maladaptive responses to other psychiatric stressors; this is unlikely to be tested. Diagnosis is always one of exclusion, and ruling out medical/psychiatric comorbidities will be key. The treatment modalities vary by disease and are unlikely to be tested. On the exam, the most important thing you will need to be able to do is simply recognize something as a somatoform disorder without confusing it for something else.

Somatoform disorders only comprised of 1%–5% of the 2016 and earlier NBMEs. While the 2017 NBME does not give an exact percentage breakdown for somatoform disorders, it is likely to have a similar number of questions. Feel free to skip to more high-yield sections if you do not have enough time to study every topic. Otherwise, prepare to spend 2–3 hours perusing this chapter.

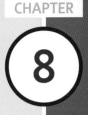

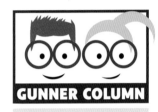

GUNNER COLUMN

A. Body Dysmorphic Disorder (BDD) (Dysmorphophobia)

Buzz Words: Obsession with body image + repeated attempts of hiding or fixing + significant impact in function → body dysmorphia

Clinical Presentation: Patients with BDD will report never being satisfied with their body image. This may manifest as excessive exercising and surgeries. The patient can also report looking in mirror frequently or asking friends constantly for validation.

PPx: None, but thought to start from bullying and teasing at a young age

MoD: Biopsychosocial, with heritability as high as 43%

Dx:

1. R/o (rule out) major depressive disorder (MDD), social phobia, and eating disorders.
2. Determine:
   (i) Muscle dysmorphia: Patient is preoccupied with body being insufficiently muscular.
   (ii) Insight specifier: how much insight patients have via their body image beliefs via the Brown Assessment of Beliefs Scale.

Tx/Mgmt:

1. Cognitive behavioral therapy (CBT) (exposure and response prevention)
2. Selective serotonin reuptake inhibitors (SSRIs)

B. Conversion Disorder (Functional Neurological Symptom Disorder)

Buzz Words: Neurologic symptoms (blindness, numbness, paralysis, "seizures") without organic/medical cause + precipitating stressor (typically emotional) + indifferent to neurologic symptoms (la belle indifference)

Clinical Presentation: Patients with conversion disorder act **indifferent** to the fact that they have some sort of neurologic dysfunction. This phenomenon is la belle indifference. No other disorder presents this way.

PPx: (1) Stress-relieving activities (yoga, meditation) while ensuring adequate treatment of psychiatric problems

MoD: Unknown, thought to be a defense mechanism that brain develops in response to threat

Dx:

1. Rule out neurologic causes from focused neurologic and medical examination (e.g.
   (i) head computed tomography/magnetic resonance imaging to r/o brain pathology;
   (ii) BMP, 3; complete blood count (CBC) 4; UA, 5; urine drug screen).
2. Rule out malingering.

Tx/Mgmt:
1. Tactful presentation of diagnosis; treat underlying issues.
2. PT/OT.
3. Treat psychiatric comorbidities.

C. Psychogenic Nonepileptic Seizures (PNES)

Buzz Words: Seizures + no electroencephalogram (EEG) findings

Clinical Presentation: Patients with seizure-like activity without EEG findings should be considered for PNES. Occurs most commonly in folks in their late teens or early 20s.

PPx: None; treat psychiatric comorbidities.

MoD: Unknown; coping mechanism as maladaptive strategy for stress.

Dx:
1. Focused physical exam
2. Video-EEG (gold-standard) to monitor patients for symptoms with concurrent EEG

Tx/Mgmt:
1. CBT
2. Selective serotonin reuptake inhibitors (SSRIs)

D. Malingering

Buzz Words: Fabricated or exaggerated symptoms (no medical evidence) + secondary gain (financial compensation, missing work, getting drugs) → malingering

Clinical Presentation: Patients who malinger on the shelf are often **nonmedical personnel** who have a clear secondary gain. Patients with factitious disorder are usually medical personnel who fake symptoms with no obvious secondary gain.

PPx: N/A

MoD: N/A

Dx:
1. Rule out psychiatric and medical comorbidities
2. Assess secondary gain

Tx/Mgmt:
1. Avoid consultations
2. Warn patients of invasive procedures
3. Psychiatric consultation or evaluation in some cases

E. Factitious Disorder (Munchausen Syndrome)

Buzz Words: Fabricated or exaggerated unrelated symptoms without cause + primary gain (attention, sympathy, leniency) + *no* psychiatric comorbidities → factitious disorder

Hypoglycemia + insulin vial found among belongings + no secondary gain → factitious disorder

QUICK TIPS
Childhood abuse is a major risk factor for psychogenic seizures.

QUICK TIPS
Never accuse a patient of malingering, no matter how sure you are.

QUICK TIPS
Secondary gain = ability to get out of obligation and stressful situation with manifested symptoms; patient is conscious of gain

QUICK TIPS
Primary gain serves to keep internal conflicts out of consciousness; expression of unacceptable feelings as physical symptoms in order to avoid dealing with them; patients are **unconscious** of their gain.

QUICK TIPS
Note that factitious disorder can *never* be diagnosed with malingering and evidence of *any* psychiatric comorbidities rules out factitious disorder.

QUICK TIPS
Note that factitious disorder can *never* be diagnosed with malingering and evidence of *any* psychiatric comorbidities rules out factitious disorder.

QUICK TIPS
Munchausen's by proxy is when another individual is used to play a patient role and usually involves a parent bringing in a "sick" child.

Clinical Presentation: There are two types of factitious disorders, and they fall into the category of somatic symptoms and related disorders. The two types of factitious disorders are *factitious disorder imposed on self* and *factitious disorder imposed on another*. Both of these conditions involve faking a medical illness (either physical or mental) in order to assume the role of the patient. In factitious disorder imposed on self, the person assumes the patient role; in factitious disorder imposed on another, the person fabricates a condition in someone under his or her care. This is most commonly seen in elderly patients or children.

Factitious disorders can be differentiated from malingering by the purpose of faking the illness. In malingering, there is a tangible gain (i.e., monetary compensation, time off work), while in factitious disorder the primary intent is psychological gain.

When faking an illness (either mental or physical) for the primary purpose of psychological gain, the person may willingly undergo unnecessary and invasive medical procedures in order to assume the role of the patient. Additionally, patients may injure themselves or inject themselves with bacteria, milk, insulin, urine, or feces. This is often seen in medical professionals, who know how to fake the condition accurately.

PPx: Protect children in Munchausen syndrome by proxy

MoD: Thought to arise from underlying personality problems leading to need for primary gain like attention and sympathy

Dx:
1. Psychiatric and medical evaluation, ruling out somatization (no intention to deceive) and conversion disorder (neurologic problem in setting of stressor) specifically

Tx/Mgmt:
1. Family therapy, support
2. Behavioral counseling

F. Hypochondriasis (Somatic Symptom Disorder)

Buzz Words: Belief of 2+ diseases for 6 months + disrupts social/occupational fxn + refuses medical advice

Clinical Presentation: Patients with hypochondriasis will believe they have an illness despite proof on the contrary. Unlike patients who malinger or have factitious disorder, hypochondriacs are often seen in the outpatient setting.

PPx: Avoid overbearing caretakers.

MoD: Hypervigilant states from other psychiatric conditions → overreaction to initial perceptions → exaggeration of symptoms to further debilitating levels

QUICK TIPS
Occupying medical facilities can cause this → White coat syndrome

Dx:
1. Rule out actual medical/psychiatric comorbidities.
2. Minimize ordering of lab tests.

Tx/Mgmt:
1. CBT
2. Schedule multiple follow-up visits

G. Pain Disorder

Buzz Words: Source of pain (i.e., accident) + psychological stressor + exaggerated pain for longer than usual

Clinical Presentation: Pain disorder is usually precipitated by a medical or anatomical reason for pain. Children suffer more from headaches and abdominal aches, adults will suffer from various symptoms with greater frequency.

PPx: N/A

MoD: Psychiatric influences exaggerate the sensation of actual pain that perpetuates

Dx:
1. R/o psychiatric comorbidities like somatization

Tx/Mgmt:
1. Psychotherapy
2. SSRIs
3. Sleep therapy

H. Somatization Disorder (Briquet Syndrome)

Buzz Words: Recurrent pain, gastrointestinal and pseudo-neurological symptoms over several years + before age 30 + unexplained by medical condition or substance use + one sexual dysfunction sign/symptom (e.g., anything related to ob/gyn such as hysteroscopy, vulvar itch)

Clinical Presentation: More recently, somatoform disorder and hypochondriasis have had their distinctions blurred. Depending on the diagnosis criteria, somatization disorder can be categorized with hypochondriasis or pain disorder, although these were initially separated in the Diagnostic and Statistical Manual of Mental Disorders, fourth edition (DSM-IV). The shelf will not expect you to be able to make these distinctions, and the differences between these diseases as they present are subtle. This being said, recognize that patients with somatization disorder are more **symptom**-focused, whereas those with hypochondriasis are more **disease**-focused. When the symptoms are almost exclusively pain, think about pain disorder.

Age: <30

> **QUICK TIPS**
> Comorbid with OCD, many patients also refuse doctors or have reassurances from many doctors.

> **QUICK TIPS**
> Somatization disorder is comorbid with many mood, anxiety, and personality disorders, and is one of the most difficult diagnoses to make clinically.

Sex: F>>M

Site of care: Outpatient

Social history: Trauma/abuse

PPx: N/A

MoD: Heightened sensitivity to internal physical sensations and pain due to chronic exposure to stressors, coping mechanism for dealing with emotional and psychological stress

Dx:

1. Rule out medical causes and make formal diagnosis when patients are <30 presenting with multiple symptoms over several years with no medical explanation

Tx/Mgmt:

1. Avoid tests and procedures if a medical workup already done
2. Reduce unnecessary drugs
3. Avoid giving sick leave
4. Single physician for care
5. **Regularly scheduled PCP visits**
6 CBT

QUICK TIPS

Somatoform = patients believe they are ill

Factitious = patients pretend they are ill

Malingering = patients pretend they are ill with external incentives

Dissociative Disorders

Dissociative disorders involve changes in identity, memory, and perception. Dissociation is a process by which individuals become temporarily detached from reality, and should be differentiated from psychosis, which is a loss of reality. Dissociation is a defense mechanism that in the case of dissociative disorders becomes pathologic and involuntary. All dissociative disorders are related to childhood history of abuse or trauma, starting usually before the age of 5. Prophylaxis is generally to treat comorbid psychiatric conditions, but is otherwise not applicable. Remember that the general mechanism for these disorders is that these are maladaptive compensatory mechanisms for dealing with stress and trauma. For the most part, all of the dissociative disorders are diagnosed by ruling out other psychiatric or medical causes, and are treated largely through a combination of behavioral therapies, eye movement desensitization and reprocessing, and rarely with anxiolytics and antidepressants. Most of the patients in clinical vignettes testing a dissociative disorder will be women, because women are far more likely to experience all dissociative disorders except depersonalization (where M = W). The most common ways you will be tested on dissociative disorders is in being able to recognize and diagnose them, while also differentiating between the various types of dissociative disorders.

A. Dissociative Identity Disorder (Multiple Personality Disorder)

Buzz Words: Trauma/abuse from childhood + two or more identities with different behavior and thinking + gaps in memory + social/occupational dysfunction → dissociative identity disorder

Clinical Presentation:

<u>Age</u>: Any

<u>Sex</u>: F>M

<u>Site of care</u>: Outpatient

<u>Social history</u>: Trauma/abuse before the age of 5

PPx: None

MoD: Compensatory mechanism for trauma in childhood

Dx: Review of history + rule out physical causes

Tx/Mgmt:

1. CBT + dialectal behavioral therapy
2. EMDR
3. SSRIs

B. Dissociative Amnesia (Psychogenic Amnesia)

Buzz Words: Occurring after stressful or traumatic periods (natural disaster, war, etc.) + unable to form memories for certain period → dissociative amnesia

Dissociative fugue: Wandering away without recollecting why → dissociative fugue

Clinical Presentation: Always remember that dissociative amnesia is not the same simple amnesia. In dissociative amnesia, memories are formed but are unlikely to be recalled, but may resurface on rare occasions. In simple amnesia, these memories are never formed in the first place and can never be recalled. Dissociative amnesia is usually transient.

PPx: N/A

MoD: Compensatory mechanism for trauma/stress related to childhood abuse

Dx: Rule out other psychiatric and medical causes

Tx/Mgmt:

1. Psychotherapy
2. CBT
3. EMDR
4. SSRIs
5. Clinical hypnosis

C. Depersonalization/Derealization Disorder (DPD)

Buzzwords:

Depersonalization: Feeling disconnected/estranged from one's bodies and thoughts + loss of control over thoughts/actions + out of body experience

Derealization: Disconnect from surroundings leading to self-harm, anxiety, panic attacks, phobias + dysfunction of social/occupational function

Clinical Presentation: Be able to differentiate depersonalization and derealization from psychosis. People with depersonalization/derealization are disconnected but always firmly are able to distinguish that their own depersonalization/derealization experiences are not reality. In psychosis, there is no distinction.

PPx: N/A

MoD: Related to severe stress + childhood trauma, inhibition of emotional experience by prefrontal cortex, with dysregulation of sympathetic fight or flight axis

Dx:

1. Psychiatric/medical history,
2. Mental status exam

Tx/Mgmt:

1. CBT
2. SSRI + benzo if DPD coincident with anxiety

QUICK TIPS

Remember that cannabis is one of the biggest causes of depersonalization/derealization.

QUICK TIPS

Depersonalization is one of the most poorly treated diseases that is often neglected by the psychiatric community

GUNNER PRACTICE

1. A 26-year-old woman who comes into your office reports not being able to move her left arm for the past 2 weeks. Her past medical history is notable for an episode of depression in her teens, but is otherwise unremarkable. Upon questioning, she reveals that she recently found out she was not offered admission to her graduate school of choice 16 days ago. Even though she is unable to move her left arm, she does not appear to be too concerned. On exam, there is no evidence for injury in her left arm, and her neurologic exam is unremarkable in other extremities. Which of the following is the most likely diagnosis?
   A. Conversion disorder
   B. Malingering
   C. Factitious disorder
   D. Hypochondriasis
   E. Psychogenic seizure

2. A 28-year-old male medical resident comes to your office for the third time in the past year asking to be worked up for Crohn disease. After a thorough physical

and history, you tell him that no organic disease is present. Despite this, he continues to test his own stool for occult bleeding and seeks further medical opinion. Which of the following is the most likely diagnosis?

A. Munchausen syndrome
B. Malingering
C. Conversion disorder
D. Hypochondriasis
E. Somatization disorder

3. An 18-year old girl is being evaluated after being accused of stabbing her uncle while he was asleep. According to her, she does not remember any of these actions, but at the same time does not feel any remorse. Her parents tell you that she has a long history of being sexually abused by her uncle. Upon questioning, her voice changes and she begins speaking rapidly, claiming she is her aunt and that she stabbed her uncle without anyone else knowing. The patient no longer responds to her real name and responds only to her aunt's name. Which of the following is the most likely diagnosis?

A. MDD with psychotic features
B. Schizophrenia
C. Dissociative fugue
D. Dissociative identity disorder
E. DPD

ANSWERS: What Would Gunner Jess/Jim Do?

1. WWGJD? A 26-year-old woman who comes into your office reports not being able to move her left arm for the past 2 weeks. Her past medical history is notable for an episode of depression in her teens, but is otherwise unremarkable. Upon questioning, she reveals that she recently found out she was not offered admission to her graduate school of choice 16 days ago. Even though she is unable to move her left arm, she does not appear to be too concerned. On exam, there is no evidence for injury in her left arm and her neurologic exam is unremarkable in other extremities. Which of the following is the most likely diagnosis?

   Answer: A. Conversion disorder

   Explanation: Neurologic signs following a precipitating stressor that appear acutely are always conversion disorder. In addition, she appears indifferent to her symptoms, which is classic for la belle difference seen in folks with conversion disorder. This should be differentiated from other somatic disorders, which often do not have precipitating stressors.

   B. Malingering → Incorrect; she has no evidence for secondary gain from not being able to move her arm. Malingering is usually not precipitated by a social stressor.

   C. Factitious disorder→ Incorrect; she has no evidence for primary gain from this, and factitious disorders are usually not precipitated by social stressors.

   D. Hypochondriasis → Hypochondriacs typically complain of having diseases without medical causes, and this leads to frequent doctor visits with normal medical exams. A diagnosis of hypochondriasis would require frequent complaints about the same problem.

   E. Psychogenic seizure → Psychogenic seizures may cause neurologic problems in the form of epilepsy, but do not usually lead to paralysis.

2. WWGJD? A 28-year-old male medical resident comes to your office for the third time in the past year asking to be worked up for Crohn disease. After a thorough physical and history, you tell him that no organic disease is present. Despite this, he continues to test his own stool for occult bleeding and seeks further medical opinion. Which of the following is the most likely diagnosis?

   Answer: D. Hypochondriasis

Explanation: Hypochondriasis is very common in those in the medical profession, known better as "white coat syndrome." Patients will have frequent complaints that they have one or more diseases, despite being constantly reassured that they have no problems.

A. Munchausen syndrome → Incorrect. There is no primary gain to be had here, and there is no evidence that this patient is attempting to be deceptive. Patients with factitious disorder are often prone to self-harm.

B. Malingering → Incorrect. There is no secondary gain to be had here, and there is no evidence that this patient is attempting to be deceptive.

C. Conversion disorder → Incorrect. There is no precipitating social stressor, nor is there a neurologic problem present.

E. Somatization disorder → Incorrect. Somatization disorder usually focuses on multiple symptoms over a long period of time without evidence for an organic cause. Whereas this patient could have somatization, his being a medical resident and complaining about a specific disease process occurring make hypochondriasis more likely.

3. WWGJD? An 18-year-old girl is being evaluated after being accused of stabbing her uncle while he was asleep. According to her, she does not remember any of these actions, but at the same time does not feel any remorse. Her parents tell you that she has a long history of being sexually abused by her uncle. Upon questioning, her voice changes and she begins speaking rapidly, claiming she is her aunt and that she stabbed her uncle without anyone else knowing. The patient no longer responds to her real name and responds only to her aunt's name. Which of the following is the most likely diagnosis?

Answer: D. Dissociative identity disorder

Explanation: A change in personality that is coincident with amnesia is typical of dissociative identity disorder. When patients take on their new identity, they are unable to form memories.

A. MDD with psychotic features → Incorrect. This patient meets no criteria for MDD based on the clinical vignette. Psychosis does not typically present with voice changes and personality changes.

B. Schizophrenia → Incorrect. This patient meets no criteria for schizophrenia, and psychosis usually occurs in the form of hearing voices, rather than through voice changes and personality changes.

C. Dissociative fugue → Incorrect. Dissociative fugue usually leads to personality changes and unintended wandering/traveling with amnesia.

E. Depersonalization disorder → Incorrect. Typically, patients with depersonalization are able to describe their experience and perceive that it is not rooted in reality. In contrast, this patient has no recollection whatsoever of their secondary identity experience.

Other Disorders/Conditions

Daniel Pustay, Leo Wang, Hao-Hua Wu, and Olga Achildi

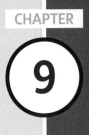

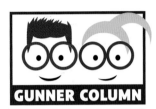

GUNNER COLUMN

This chapter covers eating and impulse control disorders, personality disorders, sexual and gender identity disorders, adverse effects of drugs, and Gunner practice (application of material). Psychiatric and personality disorders are best learned by understanding the pattern of behavior and thought exhibited. Therefore each disorder in this chapter contains a Buzz Words section, followed by a brief Clinical Presentation, Prophylaxis (PPx), Mechanism of Disease (MoD), Diagnostic Steps (Dx), and Treatment/Management (Tx/Mgmt). The diagnosis of nearly all these conditions will rely on patient history, with a few important physical signs. Little is known about the mechanism and prophylaxis of many of these disorders; however, the exam questions that come from this chapter will focus on differentiating disorders and treatment, rather than mechanism or prophylaxis.

Eating and Impulse Control Disorders

A. Anorexia Nervosa

Buzz Words: Young female + excessive dieting, exercise, or binging and purging + body mass index (BMI) less than 18.5

Clinical Presentation: Usually seen in young females who display an intense fear of gaining weight and distortion of body image. Associated symptoms include severe weight loss, lanugo, decreased bone density (osteoporosis), anemia, metatarsal stress fractures, amenorrhea (from loss of pulsatile GnRH), and electrolyte imbalances. Two subtypes:

1. Restricting type (excessive dieting)
2. Binge-eating/purging type (excessive dieting with episodes of eating large quantities of food, followed by purging, which may consist of laxatives/diuretics, vomiting, etc.)

PPx: N/A

MoD: Unknown; however, genetic factors (first-degree relative with anorexia increases risk) and psychosocial factors (societal pressures to be slender, more common in adolescents) have some implication.

Dx:
1. Patient history

Tx/Mgmt:
1. Nutritional rehabilitation (most common complication is refeeding syndrome—increased insulin leads to hypophosphatemia causing cardiac complications)
2. Psychotherapy (family therapy/group therapy)

B. Bulimia Nervosa

Buzz Words: Parotitis + enamel erosion + electrolyte imbalances + alkalosis + Russell sign (calluses on dorsal hand) + **normal BMI**

Clinical Presentation: Usually in young females who practice binge eating with inappropriate compensatory behaviors (vomiting, laxative/diuretic use, fasting, or excessive exercise). It must occur weekly for at least 3 months. In addition, it typically coexists with overvaluation of body image. Importantly, patients with bulimia nervosa maintain a normal BMI. The two subtypes are the purging type and the nonpurging type.

PPx: N/A

MoD: Unknown

Dx:
1. Patient history

Tx/Mgmt:
1. Nutritional rehabilitation
2. Psychotherapy (cognitive and behavioral)
3. Antidepressants (selective serotonin reuptake inhibitors [SSRIs]—fluoxetine)
4. Group counseling

C. Binge Eating Disorder

Buzz Words: Recurrent episodes of large food intake + feeling loss of control and guilt + no compensatory behaviors

Clinical Presentation: These patients have routine episodes of excessive, uncontrollable eating without inappropriate compensation behaviors. Feelings of loss of control, shame, distress, or guilt follow these episodes. Binge eating disorder is associated with increased risk of diabetes mellitus.

PPx: N/A

MoD: Unknown

Dx:
1. Patient history

Tx/Mgmt:
1. Psychotherapy cognitive behavioral therapy (CBT)
2. SSRI

gg AR

Cleveland Clinic Comprehensive Plan for Treatment of Eating Disorders

D. Disorders of Impulse Control

Buzz Words: Uncontrolled gambling + shoplifting + stealing + setting fires + hair pulling (bald spots)

Clinical Presentation: These include gambling, shoplifting, pyromania, and trichotillomania. In impulse control disorder, the action is preceded by a feeling of building pressure or anxiety, and then followed by a sensation of relief or happiness. The patient feels as if they cannot avoid doing actions that bring harm to themselves or others.

PPx: N/A

MoD: Unknown

Dx:

1. Patient history

Tx/Mgmt:

1. Individual or group therapy (particularly CBT)

Personality Disorders

A personality disorder is a pervasive pattern of behaviors that are chronic, inflexible, and maladaptive, which leads to distress or impaired functioning. For personality disorders, the patient is **always unaware** of the problem (no "insight"; aka ego-syntonic). On the other hand, folks who suffer from psychiatric disorders that mimic personality disorders, such as obsessive-compulsive disorder (OCD), are acutely aware of and distressed by their behavior (ego-dystonic). For diagnostic purposes, the personality trait and impairment in functioning must be relatively stable across time and situations, and they must be present by early adulthood. The best method to organize personality disorders is by cluster.

Cluster A includes paranoid, schizoid, and schizotypal personality disorders, which have a genetic link to schizophrenia. These people are perceived as odd or eccentric, without any outright psychosis, but they have difficulty developing social relationships. Remember Cluster A as "weird."

Cluster B disorders are more emotional and erratic. this cluster includes antisocial, borderline, histrionic, and narcissistic personality disorders. There is a genetic association with mood disorders and substance abuse. Remember Cluster B as "wild."

Cluster C contains avoidant, dependent, and obsessive-compulsive personality disorders (OCPD). These conditions are more anxious and fearful. Furthermore, as a group they share a genetic association with anxiety disorders. Remember Cluster C as "worried."

Questions about personality disorders will be a description of the patient's behaviors and feelings. The answer set will then require you to determine the personality disorder

QUICK TIPS
OCD = ego dystonic; OCPD = ego syntonic

QUICK TIPS
Personality disorder clusters can be remembered by "Weird, Wild, and Worried."

gg AR

Cluster A Personality Disorders Video

represented. The most important and challenging differentiation will be between disorders within a cluster. In addition to understanding the personality disorders, learn the schizophrenia spectrum (i.e., schizoid vs. schizotypal vs. schizophreniform vs. schizophrenia vs. schizoaffective), and how to differentiate between OCD and OCPD.

Personality disorders must be differentiated from the use of substances, as well as an acute onset change in mental status or behavior, which may denote a different structural or functional etiology. Exam questions rarely focus on treatment or management of personality disorders, with the only exception being dialectical behavioral therapy (DBT) for borderline personality disorder.

Cluster A

A. Paranoid Personality Disorder

Buzz Words: Mistrustful + suspicious + litigious

Clinical Presentation: This person is highly suspicious and mistrustful of others. They interpret others' motives and behaviors as malevolent, and attribute the responsibility of their own problems onto others. The main defense mechanism they use is projection. The beliefs are grounded in reality and are not considered psychotic in nature. Rarely seeks treatment, due to suspiciousness.

PPx: N/A

MoD: N/A

Dx:

  1. Patient history

Tx/Mgmt:

  1. Individual psychotherapy and anxiety/antipsychotic/antidepressant medications for associated symptoms

B. Schizoid Personality Disorder

Buzz Words: Detached + restricted emotions + lack of empathy + odd appearance + no loss of reality

Clinical Presentation: This person has limited emotional expression, and voluntarily withdraws themselves from social interactions. They are comfortable and content with their self-created isolation, and demonstrate no other thought disorders (i.e., disorganization, magical thinking, delusions, etc.). It is more common in males than females. Questions will frequently describe a male working nightshift at the post office or other isolative job settings. Also rarely seeks treatment.

PPx: N/A

MoD: N/A

Dx: Patient history

Tx/Mgmt: Individual psychotherapy and anxiety/antipsychotic/antidepressant medications for associated symptoms

C. Schizotypal Personality Disorder
Buzz Words: Peculiar or eccentric in appearance + odd thought patterns and behavior + magical thinking that is not cultural

Clinical Presentation: This person is commonly perceived as strange or unusual in appearance with magical thinking and/or ideas of reference. No outright psychosis (loss of contact with reality).

PPx: N/A

MoD: N/A

Dx:
1. Patient history

Tx/Mgmt:
1. Individual psychotherapy
2. Anxiety/antipsychotic/antidepressant medications for associated symptoms

Cluster B

D. Antisocial Personality Disorder
Buzz Words: Recurrent criminality + impulsivity, lack of empathy, and guilt + ≥18 years old

Clinical Presentation: This person has complete disregard for the safety, rights, and feelings of others as well as refusal to follow social norms. It is much more common in males than females. In order to diagnose antisocial personality disorder, the patient must be over the age of 18 (under 18 = conduct disorder), and have a history of conduct disorder before the age of 15. Commonly associated with substance use disorders.

PPx: N/A

MoD: N/A (more common in first-degree relatives and in patients of lower socioeconomic status)

Dx:
1. Patient history

Tx/Mgmt:
1. Individual psychotherapy
2. Anxiety/antipsychotic/antidepressant medications for associated symptoms

E. Borderline Personality Disorder
Buzz Words: Splitting + fear of abandonment + unstable mood and relationships + impulsive, sense of emptiness + self-mutilation

Clinical Presentation: These patients display splitting as their main defense mechanism, meaning they view everyone

gg AR

Cluster B Personality Disorders Video

as either all good or all bad. Self-mutilation and suicidal tendencies are common with these patients, sometimes for relatively trivial reasons. They report feeling bored, alone, or empty. Impulsive behaviors are very common (sex, binge eating, reckless driving, substance abuse). It is more common in females than males, and has an association with mood disorders and eating disorders. Common questions will involve young females who have recurrent suicide attempts and/or scars from wrist cutting. Patient scan may also be transiently psychotic.

PPx: N/A

MoD: N/A (five times more common in first-degree relatives)

Dx:

1. Patient history

Tx/Mgmt:

1. DBT

F. Histrionic Personality Disorder

Buzz Words: Patient who makes a scene in the waiting room + wears sexually provocative clothing + flirts with the staff or physician

Clinical Presentation: This person has excessive emotionality and excitability. They attempt to be the center of attention, dress and act in sexually provocative ways, and are overly preoccupied with superficial appearance. They cannot maintain any deep intimate relationships because they are seen as shallow, vain, and superficial.

PPx: N/A

MoD: N/A

Dx:

1. Patient history

Tx/Mgmt:

1. Individual psychotherapy
2. Anxiety/antipsychotic/antidepressant medications for associated symptoms

G. Narcissistic Personality Disorder

Buzz Words: Entitled + reacts poorly to criticism + demands the best of everything

Clinical Presentation: This person is entitled, self-centered, and grandiose; requires excessive admiration; and has no empathy for others. They have no interest in doing activities that do not directly benefit them, and react to criticism with anger or rage.

PPx: N/A

MoD: N/A

Dx:

1. Patient history

Tx/Mgmt:
1. Individual psychotherapy
2. Anxiety/antipsychotic/antidepressant medications for associated symptoms

Cluster C

H. Dependent Personality Disorder

Buzz Words: Submissive and clingy + need to be taken care of + low self-confidence + questions regard excessive romantic clinginess

Clinical Presentation: This person has an intense fear of being deserted or alone. They are submissive, passive, and obedient. They are often trapped in abusive relationships.

PPx: N/A

MoD: N/A

Dx:
1. Patient history

Tx/Mgmt:
1. Psychotherapy
2. Anxiety/antipsychotic/antidepressant medications for associated symptoms

I. Avoidant Personality Disorder

Buzz Words: Timid + low self-esteem + shy + socially inhibited

Clinical Presentation: This person is timid, socially withdrawn, and hypersensitive to rejection. Desires relationship with others, but cannot bring themselves to do it.

PPx: N/A

MoD: N/A

Dx:
1. Patient history

Tx/Mgmt:
1. Psychotherapy
2. Anxiety/antipsychotic/antidepressant medications for associated symptoms

J. Obsessive-Compulsive Personality Disorder

Buzz Words: Perfectionist + inflexible + fails to meet deadlines due to preoccupation with details + ego syntonic

Clinical Presentation: This person is preoccupied with order, perfection, and control, which makes them stubborn and indecisive. Applies broadly to all areas of life, whereas in OCD the obsessions/compulsions are specific. It is more commonly seen in males than females. Importantly, their behavior is ego-syntonic (consistent within one's beliefs). Patients with OCPD do not think anything is wrong with them, whereas patients with OCD know that something is wrong.

PPx: N/A

MoD: N/A

Dx:

1. Patient history

Tx/Mgmt:

1. Psychotherapy and anxiety/antipsychotic/ antidepressant medications for associated symptoms

Sexual and Gender Identity Disorders

A. Gender Identity Disorder

Buzz Words: Parents bring in child who prefers to play with toys of opposite gender + dress as opposite gender

Clinical Presentation: This patient has strong and persistent cross-gender identification. This leads to discomfort with sex assigned at birth, leading to impaired functioning or significant distress. Distinct from sexuality, which describes a person's attraction preferences.

PPx: N/A

MoD: Differential exposure to prenatal sex hormones (increased androgen levels in females, decreased androgen levels in males, leading to anatomical changes in hypothalamic nuclei)

Dx:

1. Diagnosed through patient interview, typically in children

Tx/Mgmt:

1. Assist the parents/family members to accept the person as they are, because gender at school age is permanent
2. CBT, hormone therapy, and/or surgery

B. Psychosexual Dysfunction

Buzz Words: Loss of sexual interest/fantasies + arousal inhibition + orgasmic inhibition + pain with sex

Clinical Presentation: The inability to become aroused or achieve sexual satisfaction for psychological reasons. Sexual dysfunctions may be primary (always present), or secondary (after a period of normal functioning). For diagnosis, they must be differentiated from medication effects, physical causes, and medical illnesses. This category includes a variety of conditions, including:

Sexual desire disorders (hypoactive sexual desire or sexual aversion)

Sexual arousal disorders (erectile dysfunction)

Orgasmic disorders (anorgasmia, premature ejaculation)

Sexual pain disorders (dyspareunia, vaginismus)

PPx: N/A

MoD: Psychological causes of sexual dysfunction may be a result of stress, relationship problems, anxiety, or depression

Dx:

1. Rule out (r/o) external causes. Differential may include medications (antihypertensives, neuroleptics, SSRIs, ethanol), diseases (diabetes mellitus, STIs), and psychological etiologies (performance anxiety, depression)
2. For erectile dysfunction, psychological etiology is determined by absence of nighttime tumescence.

Tx/Mgmt: May be behavioral, medical, or surgical, depending on etiology

1. Behavioral: sensate-focus exercises (used for sexual desire, arousal, and orgasmic disorders), squeeze technique (used for premature ejaculation), relaxation/hypnosis/systemic desensitization (reduce disorder associated with sexual performance), psychotherapy (management of underlying mood or emotional disorder)
2. Medical: SSRIs (used to delay orgasm for premature ejaculation), opioid antagonists and vasodilators (have been used to manage erectile disorder); sildenafil citrate (Viagra), vardenafil (Levitra/Nuviva), tadalafil (Cialis) (used to stop phosphodiesterase-5, which increases cGMP concentration, thus vasodilating the vessels in the penis, causing erection); vasodilator injections (papaverine/phentolamine); and apomorphine hydrochloride (increases dopamine in the brain, causing increased sexual interest and erectile function)
3. Surgical: prosthetic devices (used to manage erectile dysfunction)

Adverse Effects of Drugs

A. Steroid Induced Psychosis

Buzz Words: Psychosis + child with asthma exacerbation recently put on steroids or adults with disorders controlled on steroids that have a change in mental status

Clinical Presentation: This includes the traditional signs and symptoms of psychosis seen in patients with recent administration of glucocorticoids, or on high doses of glucocorticoids over an extended period. Opposing symptoms for patients; some experience euphoria, hypomania, anxiety, akathisia, depression, and emotional lability.

PPx: N/A

MoD: Not completely understood; administration is associated with decreased corticotrophin, NE and beta-endorphin in cerebrospinal fluid, and increased glutamate concentration leading to neuronal toxicity.

Dx:

1. Patient history, timing of drug administration to change in mental status

Tx/Mgmt:

1. Decrease/discontinue dosage of glucocorticoids
2. If symptoms persist, begin antipsychotic treatment

B. Drug-Induced Psychogenic Polydipsia

Buzz Words: Hyponatremia + confusion + lethargy + psychosis + seizures

Clinical Presentation: This is when a medication causes a person to drink excessive amounts of water, which may lead to water intoxication and hyponatremia. Can be fatal.

PPx: N/A

MoD: Multifactorial, likely due to change in hypothalamic thirst center as primary cause. Commonly from diuretics, antipsychotics, antidepressants, anticonvulsants, and chemotherapeutic agents

Dx:

1. Patient history (distinguish cause of polydipsia)
2. BMP with hyponatremia or other electrolyte imbalance

Tx/Mgmt:

1. Fluid restriction
2. Medication alteration

C. Varenicline and Suicide

Buzz Words: Patient attempting to quit smoking + using varenicline (Chantix) + asking about the risks of such medications

Clinical Presentation: On the shelf, will present as suicidal patient recently prescribed varenicline

PPx: N/A

MoD: N/A

Dx:

1. Patient history

Tx/Mgmt:

1. Change smoking cessation strategy

GUNNER PRACTICE

1. A 20-year-old college student presents to her primary care physician for a well-visit check-up. She works in the library sorting returned books. She spends most of her time reading, and on the weekends prefers to go on long hikes instead of socializing with classmates. She is studying English and generally receives good grades. She says that she is invited to go out with classmates, but she always refuses because she thinks they won't like her. This behavior is most similar to which personality disorder?

A. Schizotypal personality disorder
B. Schizoid personality disorder
C. Antisocial personality disorder
D. Histrionic personality disorder
E. Avoidant personality disorder

2. A 16-year-old female high school student comes to the physician because of swelling and pain on her cheek near her ear. She has a BMI of 17, pulse of 89, blood pressure of 115/65, and temperature of 98 degrees Fahrenheit. Upon questioning, she reveals that she tries to eat only healthy foods, but she cannot keep it under control. She states that some nights she goes out to eat several meals from a fast food restaurant, and then feels guilty once she has finished them. On physical exam, the physician notes calluses on the back of her right hand. This behavior most closely suggests

A. Anorexia nervosa restricting type
B. Obsessive compulsive personality disorder
C. Anorexia nervosa binge-eating/purging type
D. Histrionic personality disorder
E. Bulimia nervosa binge-eating/purging type

3. A 45-year-old medical assistant faints in the parking lot of the hospital. She reports that she has experienced similar episodes in the past, and her records show three events at different offices in the last 2 years. After she is brought into the emergency department, her vital signs are pulse of 85, blood pressure of 123/68, temperature of 97.5 degrees Fahrenheit, oxygen saturation of 99% in room air. Her history shows no other episodes of lightheadedness or dizziness, no shaking or tremors were witnessed, and she is alert and oriented to time, place, and person. Her laboratory studies show hypoglycemia, hyperinsulinemia, normal sodium levels, and a depressed plasma C-peptide. Which does this clinical scenario most likely represent?

A. Malingering
B. Diabetes mellitus
C. Factitious disorder
D. Conversion disorder
E. Narcolepsy

ANSWERS: What Would Gunner Jess/Jim Do?

1. **WWGJD?** A 20-year-old college student presents to her primary care physician for a well-visit check-up. She works in the library sorting returned books. She spends most of her time reading, and on the weekends prefers to go on long hikes instead of socializing with classmates. She is studying English, and generally receives good grades. She says that she is invited to go out with classmates, but she always refuses because she thinks they won't like her. This behavior is most similar to which personality disorder?

   Answer: E. Avoidant personality disorder

   Explanation: Patient voluntarily isolates herself socially, for fear of being disliked or rejected. She desires to be social, but chooses to remain alone. She chose a job that allows her to avoid social contact with others, and plans her activities to maintain her isolation.

   A. Schizotypal personality disorder → Incorrect. In order for this to be correct, the question would need to describe magical thinking, ideas of reference, or an eccentric personality or appearance.

   B. Schizoid personality disorder → Incorrect. This answer can be ruled out because although both schizoid and avoidant personality disorders have social isolation, this patient wishes to have more friends and social contact. This behavior is more characteristic of an avoidant personality disorder, whereas a person with schizoid personality disorder would not be interested in making more friends.

   C. Antisocial personality disorder → Incorrect. This answer refers to a person with disregard for the safety, well-being, or feelings of others. They are generally aggressive, impulsive, and sometimes malicious. This patient does not exhibit any of these behaviors or feelings, and does not have a history of conduct disorder as a child.

   D. Histrionic personality disorder → Incorrect. This answer choice describes a person that is dramatic, attention seeking, and provocative. This patient is not attention-seeking, and her personality is better described by her social isolation.

2. **WWGJD?** A 16-year-old female high school student comes to the physician because of swelling and pain on her cheek near her ear. She has a BMI of 17, pulse of

89, blood pressure of 115/65, and a temperature of 98 degrees Fahrenheit. Upon questioning, she reveals that she tries to eat only healthy foods, but she cannot keep it under control. She states that some nights she goes out to eat several meals from a fast food restaurant, and then feels guilty once she has finished them. On physical exam, the physician notes calluses on the back of her right hand. This behavior most closely suggests

Answer: C. Anorexia nervosa binge-eating/purging type.

Explanation: The cheek swelling and pain describes parotitis, a common symptom in patients that purge using self-induced vomiting. The calluses on the back of the hand (Russell sign) reinforce this purging practice. The trips to get fast food describe instances of bingeing, and the BMI of 17 point toward anorexia nervosa as a better answer than bulimia nervosa.

A. Anorexia nervosa restricting type → Incorrect. This patient's physical findings of parotitis and Russell sign show that she has binge-eating/purging type rather than restricting type of anorexia nervosa.

B. Obsessive compulsive personality disorder → Incorrect. This question does not describe any perfectionist mannerisms, and instead focuses on the eating behaviors and physical finding of the patient.

D. Histrionic personality disorder → Incorrect. These patients typically desire to be the center of attention; they are provocative, dramatic, and flirtatious. This patient does not show any of those signs.

E. Bulimia nervosa binge-eating/purging type → Incorrect. Although this question does describe a binge-eating/purging type of eating disorder, because this patient has a BMI less than 18.5, she fits better into anorexia nervosa than bulimia nervosa.

3. WWGJD? A 45-year-old medical assistant faints in the parking lot of the hospital. She reports that she has experienced similar episodes in the past, and her records show three events at different offices in the last 2 years. After she is brought into the Emergency Department, her vital signs are: pulse of 85, blood pressure of 123/68, temperature of 97.5 degrees Fahrenheit, oxygen saturation is 99% in room air. Her history shows no other episodes of lightheadedness or dizziness, no

shaking or tremors were witnessed, and she is alert and oriented to time, place, and person. Her **laboratory studies show hypoglycemia, hyperinsulinemia, normal sodium levels, and a depressed plasma C-peptide.** Which does this clinical scenario most likely represent?

Answer: C. Factitious disorder

Explanation: This question describes a patient with factitious disorder, a condition in which the patient fakes a medical or mental illness for the primary purpose of receiving medical attention or assuming the patient role. This patient fainted after injecting herself with insulin in the hospital parking lot. This is evident by the increased insulin and decreased plasma C-peptide concentrations. People who have factitious disorder often worked in the medical field in some capacity and understand how to simulate the illness believably.

A. Malingering → Incorrect. Malingering is feigning an illness in order to receive some tangible gain. This question does not describe the patient's purpose to gain any compensation; therefore malingering is not the best option.

B. Diabetes mellitus → Incorrect. This answer is incorrect because of the laboratory values, which point toward exogenous insulin used to cause hypoglycemia and therefore the fainting episode.

D. Conversion disorder → Incorrect. This disorder describes a sudden and dramatic loss of sensation or motor function, typically after a very stressful event. The question does not describe any ongoing neurological deficits in the patient.

E. Narcolepsy → Incorrect. This question does not describe a typical sleep attack; rather it is a fainting episode, which is followed by the laboratory values indicating exogenous insulin use.

Disease of Nervous System and Special Senses

Hao-Hua Wu, Leo Wang, and Olga Achildi

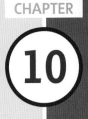
Introduction

Contrary to popular medical student opinion, the neurology section is very well represented on the psychiatry shelf; out of 110 questions, 10%–15% will focus primarily on neurological disorders such as Parkinson disease, narcolepsy, or absence seizures. Thus you should resist the urge to skip or skim this chapter, particularly if you have not done your neurology rotation yet. Focus on the symptoms and drugs that overlap with other psychiatric conditions (e.g., hallucinations in Lewy body dementia, mood stabilizers used to treat seizures). Also, make sure you understand the organizing principle behind groups of disorders, such as the role of the basal ganglia in movement disorders. Understanding the big picture behind these neurological concepts will help you for every single shelf exam.

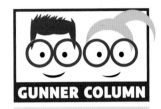

GUNNER COLUMN

This chapter is divided into six sections: (1) global cerebral dysfunction, (2) degenerative disorders/amnestic syndromes, (3) movement disorders, (4) sleep disorders, (5) seizure disorders, and (6) Gunner practice. There are a few congenital diseases, such as fetal alcohol syndrome, that fall into the "Diseases of Nervous System and Special Senses" category; these are covered in Chapter 3.

Global Cerebral Dysfunction

For the psychiatry shelf, disorders stemming from global cerebral dysfunction are frequently tested because there is a lot of overlap between specialties. Delirium, for example, can be evaluated and treated by psychiatrists, neurologists, internists, and even surgeons. Disorders of global cerebral dysfunction can also imitate other disease processes. For instance, it is important to be familiar with how to differentiate delirium from psychosis (e.g., psychosis = normal electroencephalography (EEG); delirium = abnormal EEG) and dementia (e.g. delirium = waxes and wanes; dementia = persistent).

A. Delirium

Buzz Word: Fluctuating mental status (vs. dementia which is persistent) + sundowning (worse at night) + acute onset + impaired consciousness + visual hallucinations

Clinical Presentation: Patients with delirium present with agitation, hallucinations, tremulousness, incoherent thought, distracted, and disoriented. They frequently have prior alcohol/sedative drug use (looking for delirium in setting of withdrawal).

PPx: (1) Let patient sleep through night (no 5 a.m. labs), (2) stop unnecessary meds, (3) decrease stimuli, (4) orient patient to room with calendar and clock

MoD: Caused by many medical insults, including alcohol withdrawal, hypoxemia, intracranial bleeding, infection (both sepsis and primary brain infections), medications (anticholinergics, benzos)

Dx:

1. Clinical
2. UA/UCx, glucose, BMP, blood cultures, RPR to rule out (r/o) possible etiologies
3. Computed tomography/magnetic resonance imaging (CT/MRI) to r/o structural abnormalities
4. EEG (to r/o seizure), but if taken will show diffuse background slowing (vs. psychosis, which has a normal EEG)
5. Medication review (polypharmacy)

Tx/Mgmt:

1. Delirium PPx (e.g., let patient sleep, stop unnecessary meds, decrease stimuli, orient patient with calendar and clock)
2. Haloperidol, quetiapine for acute agitation
3. **Avoid benzos** in the **elderly**, although can be given in young patients

B. Amnestic Disorder

Buzz Words: Isolated amnesia + underlying medical condition + immediately postop + benzos during surgery + can't learn new information or recall old + confabulation

Clinical Presentation: See Buzz Words

PPx: Avoid precipitating meds like benzos

MoD: Meds (e.g., benzos) + trauma + tumor + alcohol + multiple sclerosis

Dx:

1. Medical work up (look for electrolyte abnormalities)
2. Urine drug screen (UDS) to look for medications
3. CT/MRI to look for structural lesion

Tx/Mgmt: None

C. Transient Global Amnesia

Buzz Words: Amnesia + can't learn new info + lasts several hours + **personal identity remains intact**

QUICK TIPS

Electrolyte imbalance like hypercalcemia may cause delirium. Make sure you know how to calculate corrected calcium, since increased albumin in the body may make the calcium reading on the complete metabolic panel artificially low. Corrected calcium = (0.8 * [Normal Albumin − Pt's Albumin]) + Serum Ca

Clinical Presentation: The key to identifying transient global amnesia is to recognize that personal identity remains intact. On the other hand, dissociative fugue patients lose their personal identification. The chief complaint is normal behavior with amnesia (may manifest as repetitive questioning) and consciousness remains normal. May be associated with history of migraines.

PPx: Avoid precipitating insult (such as benzos)

MoD: Unknown, but similar presentation could result from focal seizure, transient ischemic event, migraine

Dx:

1. Medical workup (look for electrolyte abnormality)
2. UDS to look for medications
3. EEG to rule out seizure
4. CT/MRI to look for structural lesion

Tx/Mgmt: None; patients almost always recover spontaneously

Degenerative Disorders/Amnestic Syndromes

Out of the 10–15 neurology questions you will get on the psych shelf, most of them will come from degenerative disorders, which include Alzheimer, Huntington, or dementia. This is the case because the presenting symptoms may sometimes be similar to psychiatric disease (e.g., Lilliputian hallucinations in Lewy body dementia). From a practical standpoint, psychiatry consults are frequently called for patients with degenerative neurologic disorders to assess decision-making capacity (see Chapter 2).

The degenerative neurological disorders predominantly refer to diseases that lead to dementia (i.e., a progressive decline in cognition, language, memory, or personality). Although there is significant overlap in the clinical presentation of dementias, the presenting symptoms may offer clues to the underlying cause. Alzheimer disease tends to first cause memory loss, frontotemporal dementia initially causes personality changes, and Lewy body dementia exhibits Parkinsonian signs. The clinical presentations often correspond to the brain regions most impacted by disease (i.e., frontotemporal dementia will show changes in behavior and dramatic atrophy of the frontal lobes). The underlying pathology for most of these disorders is based on the accumulation and spread of abnormally folded proteins, such as beta-amyloid plaques and abnormal tau protein phosphorylation in Alzheimer disease.

While the degenerative dementias are irreversible, a similar clinical picture can result from reversible causes

QUICK TIPS

Dementia = persistent/progressive decline in intellectual/cognitive function with preserved consciousness

99 AR

Organizing Chart for Dementias

99 AR

Radiological Correlates of Dementia

(dementia due to treatable conditions). The most commonly tested reversible causes of dementia include hypothyroidism, human immunodeficiency virus (HIV), neurosyphilis, vitamin B12 deficiency, Wernicke-Korsakoff (alcohol related), normal pressure hydrocephalus (NPH), and infectious etiologies (like Cryptococcus and Lyme disease). A common workup to exclude reversible causes of dementia includes a CT/MRI, lumbar puncture, RPR for syphilis, and vitamin B12 and TSH levels. Screening for HIV and measurement of copper levels (Wilson disease), cortisol (Cushing's), and heavy metal concentrations may also be warranted with the appropriate clinical history. For the purpose of the psychiatry shelf, however, just focus on the conditions most relevant, such as HIV-associated dementia and NPH.

The degenerative neurological diseases will be organized based on their most common presenting symptom. Since the presenting symptoms relate to the underlying pathology and distribution of disease, this approach provides a framework for organizing the different diseases during study.

Memory Loss as the Predominant Symptom

A. Alzheimer Disease

Buzz Words: Older individual + progressive forgetfulness (short-term memory loss) + chronic and progressive + word-finding difficulties + <24 on MMSE + apraxia + aphasia + agnosia + impairs ADLs (vs. mild cognitive impairment or normal aging) → Alzheimer dementia

Pseudodementia is the term used for dementia patients who present with depressive symptomatology early in disease course. This is frequently tested on the shelf and should be thought of as an early manifestation of dementia rather than its own separate disease. Make sure to perform an MMSE on patients with depression and memory loss.

Clinical Presentation: Patients with Alzheimer disease are typically >60 years old and present with reduction in short-term memory (unable to remember newly learned facts) and word-finding difficulty. Paranoia, personality changes, and executive dysfunction may also be prominent. Women have 3 times increased prevalence compared with men. If Down syndrome is present in past medical history, symptoms will present much earlier in the lifespan.

PPx: None

MoD: Mediated by amyloid beta plaques (extracellular) and neurofibrillary tangles (intracellular)

Widespread neuronal loss and atrophy, prominent in the temporal lobe and extending to the frontal lobes, parietal lobes, the nucleus basalis of Meynert (cholinergic; see below for therapeutic implications)

Down syndrome increases the risk of developing Alzheimer's (because amyloid beta protein precursor is located on chromosome 21)

Familial types—mutations of genes of APP and presenilin-1 protein (PSEN-1) and presenilin-2 protein (PSEN-2) that can lead to abnormal amyloid peptide accumulation

Dx:
1. MMSE
2. R/o reversible causes of dementia by looking at TSH, T3, T4, or B12 levels, RPR for syphilis
3. Head MRI to r/o structural lesions will show diffuse atrophy/enlarged ventricles with disproportionate atrophy of the hippocampus

Tx/Mgmt:
1. Donepezil (acetylcholinesterase inhibitor)
2. Galantamine, rivastigmine (acetylcholinesterase [AChe] inhibitors)
3. For moderate or severe → Memantine (N-methyl-d-aspartate [NMDA] antagonist)

Antipsychotics, such as olanzapine and quetiapine, are sometimes used to control psychosis, aggression, and agitation that may develop.

> **FOR THE WARDS**
> As with the other neurodegenerative causes of dementia, the diagnosis cannot be definitive unless an autopsy is performed.

Behavioral and Personality Changes as the Predominant Symptom

B. Frontotemporal Dementia (FTD, aka Pick Disease)

Buzz Words: Inappropriate behavior/poor judgment + personality changes + disinhibition + hypersexuality + snout reflex + intraneuronal silver staining inclusions (tau bodies aka Pick's bodies) or TDP-43 inclusions

Clinical Presentation: Frontal temporal dementia is the second most common cause of early onset dementia (after Alzheimer). On the shelf, it is can be identified as a patient with memory difficulties who is disinhibited (e.g., says things that are uncharacteristically offensive). It presents in patients more than 55 years old, with the chief complaint being one of two variants: behavioral and language.

Behavioral variant = Personality changes predominate; apathy, disinhibition, perseveration, eating disorders; insight is impaired.

Language variant = Aphasias and apraxias are predominant early symptoms.

A significant number of FTLD patients will also have signs of motor neuron disease (amyotrophic lateral sclerosis [ALS] is also caused by TDP-43 inclusions).

PPx: None

MoD: Severe atrophy of the frontal and temporal lobes secondary to

Tau protein inclusions OR

TDP-43 protein inclusions

Dx:

1. MMSE, neurobehavioral assessment
2. CT/MRI → show disproportionate atrophy of frontal/temporal lobes
3. R/o reversible dementia (thyroid, B12)

Note: As with the other neurodegenerative causes of dementia, the diagnosis cannot be definitive unless an autopsy is performed.

Tx/Mgmt:

1. Only symptomatic treatment is currently available (no Food and Drug Administration approved drug)
2. Olanzapine/antipsychotic for severe disinhibition, aggression, and agitation

Movement Disorder as the Predominant Symptom

C. Lewy Body Dementia (LBD)

Buzz Words: Lilliputian hallucinations (benign, **small** hallucinations) + episodic confusion + impaired visuospatial function + dementia less than 12 months after onset of bradykinesia, tremor, abnormal posture, rigidity

Clinical Presentation: LBD is high yield because of its distinct Buzz Words in the setting of memory loss (e.g., Lilliputian hallucinations). If dementia more than 12 months, Parkinson disease with dementia (discussed later). Patients present with Parkinsonian symptoms (bradykinesia, tremor, abnormal posture, rigidity) and dementia (dementia may precede or follow Parkinsonian symptoms).

Visual hallucinations and rapid eye movement (REM) **sleep behavior** disorders often seen

PPx: None

MoA: Intracytoplasmic alpha-synuclein inclusions diffusely seen throughout the cortex and substantia nigra—leads to degeneration of dopamine releasing neurons

Dx:

1. Clinical exam and history demonstrating Parkinsonian syndrome, recurrent hallucinations, REM sleep behavior disorders, and dementia

One clue to diagnosis is extreme sensitivity to neuroleptics—confusion, neuroleptic malignant syndrome, worsening Parkinson symptoms

Tx/Mgmt:

1. Treat parkinsonian features with levo-carbidopa (but may lead to worsening hallucinations/delirium)

2. Treat cognitive symptoms with acetylcholinesterase inhibitors (Donepezil)

Dopaminergic agonists often trigger visual hallucinations and psychotic behaviors.

Hypersensitivity to antipsychotics

D. Parkinson Disease (PD)

Buzz Words: Cogwheel rigidity + resting tremor + shuffling gait + bradykinesia + postural instability + micrographia + respond to levodopa + dementia after 12 months

Clinical Presentation: PD is the second most common neurodegenerative disease (after Alzheimer) and is caused by the deposition of alpha-synuclein in the pigmented nuclei of the brainstem. The shelf exam will test your ability to recognize the diagnostic features of Parkinson's and the available therapies. In addition, PD patients sometimes develop dementia, and some patients with Parkinson symptoms develop dementia very early in their disease course. These patients will have more widespread alpha-synuclein deposition and be diagnosed with Lewy body dementia. Parkinson's can also be considered a **hypo**kinetic movement disorder.

The chief complaint will likely be one of four complaints: bradykinesia, resting tremor, postural instability, cogwheel rigidity. There is a possible link to repeated head trauma and organophosphate exposure may increase risk (toxic to dopaminergic substantia nigra neurons).

PPx: None

MoD: Lewy bodies (alpha-synuclein aggregates) accumulate in brainstem pigmented nuclei (including substantia nigra) → Leads to neuronal death and loss of dopaminergic neurons in substantia nigra

The bradykinesia is secondary to loss of dopaminergic neurons in the substantia nigra. The direct pathway receives less activation (so indirect > direct). → Movement is difficult to initiate.

Dx:

1. Clinical exam with resting "pill rolling" tremor, bradykinesia, rigidity
2. MRI/CT to rule out mimics of Parkinson's
3. Favorable response with levodopa
4. DaTSCAN (SPECT scan using dopamine transporter labeled tracer; detection of dopamine uptake deficiency in caudate and putamen)

Normal pressure hydrocephalus may mimic the gait and postural instability of Parkinson's and can be treated with an LP.

> **QUICK TIPS**
>
> Postural instability = loss of reflexes that maintain posture (leads to falls)

Essential tremor (ET) may be confused with PD, but the ET tremor is made worse with **action** and the PD tremor is worse at **rest**.

Progressive supranuclear palsy (PSP) may present with rigidity and falls (instability), but has a vertical gaze palsy.

Parkinson symptoms and dementia occurring at roughly the same time should bring up Lewy body dementia.

Tx/Mgmt: Treatment cannot reverse the alpha-synuclein pathology, but focuses on symptom management.

1. Levodopa-carbidopa → replaces dopamine lost with damage of substantia nigra
   - Carbidopa is a decarboxylase inhibitor (prevents degradation of levodopa before it gets to the brain).
   - COMT inhibitors are also used with levodopa to extent plasma half-life (COMT degrades levodopa).
   - Main side effect is dyskinesias → involuntary jerking movements
2. MAO-B inhibitors (rasagiline, selegiline) may improve motor symptoms alone or complement the effects of levodopa. MAO-B breaks down dopamine in the central nervous system
3. Dopamine agonists (bromocriptine, pramipexole) → direct effect of effect on striatal neurons; less potent than levodopa. Main side effects are hypotension and hallucinations/confusion
4. Anticholinergic agents (benztropine) → tremor reduction, less impact on bradykinesia
5. Deep brain stimulation if medication fails. Electrodes inhibit subthalamic nucleus (indirect pathways)

99 AR

Mechanisms of Parkinson Therapies

E. Progressive Supranuclear Palsy (aka Steele-Richardson-Olszewski Syndrome)

Buzz Words: Unable to look down without moving neck + progressive rigidity + dementia + pseudobulbar (lips/tongue/pharyngeal/laryngeal muscles) palsy

Clinical Presentation: Identifying patients with PSP is typically straightforward: look for patients who are unable to move their eyes in the vertical direction in the setting of dementia. The chief complaint may be unsteady gait/imbalance with development of ocular signs (loss of voluntary vertical movements), dystonia of neck muscles, slurred speech, and dysphagia.

99 AR

Clinical Features of Progressive Supranuclear Palsy

PPx: None

MoD: Idiopathic, but neurons in basal ganglia and brainstem are seen to degenerate with phosphorylated tau present

Dx:

1. Clinical exam to differentiate from Parkinson's (looking for ocular palsies/dystonia/pseudobulbar signs)
2. MRI may show atrophy of midbrain (in late cases)

Tx/Mgmt:

1. Supportive care
2. Levodopa only slightly effective for rigidity/akinesia
3. Benztropine/botulin injections for dystonia

F. Huntington Disease (HD)

Buzz Words: Atrophy of the caudate nucleus + forgetfulness + family history of early death + change in personality + chorea + depression

Clinical Presentation: HD is the most high-yield disorder of this chapter, given how frequently it appears on multiple shelf exams. It is an autosomal dominant condition caused by CAG repeat expansions in the *huntingtin* gene. Patients exhibit wild jerking movements (chorea) and dementia as its prominent features. Many patients develop depression, and the suicide rate is quite high. No effective therapies exist. HD can also be considered a hyperkinetic movement disorder. The patient's chief complaint may be personality changes emerge first (depression, impulsivity, irritability), diminished attention/concentration, with preserved memory. Patients can also appear "fidgety" with later development of widespread chorea. There is a family history of chorea/early death. The disease manifests at younger age with each generation (anticipation, as explained later).

PPx: (1) Genetic testing for counseling

MoD: CAG repeats in Huntington gene on chromosome 4 expand during replication → increasing lengths = more severe/younger onset of disease → CAG expansion = expansion of polyglutamine region of Huntington protein → proteins aggregate in neuron nuclei → loss of GABA and ACh containing neurons in basal ganglia → atrophy of caudate and putamen

The mutant huntingtin protein may also interrupt transcriptional proteins or sensitize cells to glutamate excitotoxicity

Dx:

1. Family history with genetic testing for CAG repeats (>39)
2. CT/MRI with atrophy of caudate/putamen and enlarged ventricles

QUICK TIPS

Anticipation = earlier onset in successive generations. During meiosis the CAG repeats can expand so children may have longer expansions than the parents.

 AR

Caudate Atrophy in HD

Tx/Mgmt: Treatment focuses on controlling the chorea:
1. Haloperidol (dopamine antagonist)
2. Tetrabenazine/reserpine (decrease dopamine release as VMAT inhibitors)
3. Antidepressants for depression/suicidality

Neurodegenerative Disorders Secondary to Systemic Conditions

G. Vascular Dementia

Buzz Words: Sudden, stepwise decrease in memory/cognition + focal neurologic findings

Clinical Presentation: Patients with vascular dementia are >40 years old and exhibit cognitive decline (dementia) that advances stroke by stroke (stepwise). Risk factors for stroke (high blood pressure, diabetes, atrial fibrillation).

PPX: (1) Stroke prevention (aspirin, statin, anticoag for AFb), (2) risk factors include HTN, AFb, CAD

MoD: Caused by ischemic/hemorrhagic infarcts in multiple brain areas (thalami, basal ganglia, brainstem, cortex)

Dx:
1. MMSE with temporal association between cognitive decline and strokes
2. Rule out reversible causes of dementia
3. CT/MRI shows multiple lesions of cortex/subcortical structures

Tx/Mgmt: Treatment focuses on preventing recurrent strokes (discussed previously)

H. HIV-Associated Dementia (aka HIV-Associated Neurocognitive Disorder)

Buzz Words: Progressive cognitive problems, including memory loss + immunocompromised young adult + neutropenia + acute onset of symptoms

Clinical Presentation: On the psychiatry shelf, patients with HIV (or AIDS-defining illnesses like pneumocystis jiroveci pneumonia) and memory issues should be considered to have HIV-associated dementia until proven otherwise. It is a later stage complication of HIV that presents as subacute progressive dementia with decreased memory and attention, apathy, incoordination of limbs, ataxic gait.

PPx: (1) Treatment of HIV with HAART

MoD: Diffuse rarefaction (decreased density) of cerebral white matter → may be direct result of infection by HIV

Dx:
1. CD4 count
2. CBC
3. CT/MRI to r/o PML

Tx/Mgmt:
1. HAART

I. Normal Pressure Hydrocephalus

Buzz Words: Has difficulty walking + urinary incontinence + mental decline

Clinical Presentation: The NPH triad is wet (urinary incontinence), wobbly (cannot walk; so-called magnetic gait or gait apraxia), and weird (memory loss). Since this is such a frequently tested topic for the neuro shelf, the test writers get **very creative** when it comes to describing these three symptoms. For instance, a patient's relative could describe the patient as "hasn't been able to hold it in recently" and one would have to ascertain the "wet" symptom of the triad.

PPx: None

MoD: Defective superior sagittal sinus → clogged arachnoid granulations → communicating hydrocephalus → stretching of the corona radiata (descending cortical tracts)

Dx:
1. CT
2. LP (likely show normal pressure cerebrospinal fluid)

Tx/Mgmt:
1. Serial LPs (symptoms drastically improve with high-volume spinal tap)
2. Ventriculoperitoneal shunting

MNEMONIC

Wet, wobbly, and weird = NPH

FOR THE WARDS

NPH usually has normal cerebrospinal fluid on LP, but recent data suggest it maybe intermittently elevated.

Movement Disorders

Movement disorders refer to diseases that result in either too much movement (hyperkinetic) or too little movement (hypokinetic). The only hypokinetic disorder that will be discussed is PD, described earlier by bradykinesia, rigidity, resting tremor, and postural instability. The hyperkinetic disorders include HD ("Global Cerebral Dysfunction"), essential tremor, acute dystonia, and Tourette syndrome. The distinction between hypokinetic and hyperkinetic disorders is not perfect (i.e., both essential tremor and Parkinson's are both characterized by tremor), but refers to the overall clinical picture.

The main player when it comes to movement disorders is the basal ganglia, a collection of different nuclei connected through several circuits. It includes the caudate and putamen (together called the striatum), the globus pallidus, the subthalamic nucleus, and the substantia nigra. Running within the basal ganglia are two pathways: the direct pathway and the indirect pathway. Put simply, activation of the direct pathway allows the motor cortex to initiate movement, and activation of the indirect pathway prevents movement. Activation of the direct pathway and inactivation of the indirect pathway can be achieved with dopamine from the substantia nigra, which connects with neurons in the striatum (caudate and putamen). We can now explain two important disorders. In Parkinson's, diseased cells in the substantia nigra are destroyed, so less dopamine is released. This means that the direct pathway is less activated, and the indirect pathway is less inactivated (or more activated!). The balance is tipped toward the indirect pathway and movement becomes difficult to initiate. In Huntington disease, the indirect pathway neurons in the striatum are damaged. This leads to an imbalance in favor of the direct pathway and wild, jerky movements.

A. Essential Tremor

Buzz Words: Symmetrical action tremor of the hands + quivering of the voice (vocal tremor) + difficulty with precise tasks (threading needle) + better with alcohol/propranolol

Clinical Presentation: Essential tremor (ET, benign tremor, or familial tremor) is the most common type of tremor. It commonly affects the arms and is worsened with movement (action tremor). Alcohol diminishes the tremor and anxiety; exercise and fatigue make it worse. The tremor is often familial, exhibiting an autosomal dominant inheritance pattern. ET should be distinguished from an intention tremor, which is caused by cerebellar dysfunction and presents when reaching for an object. Intention tremors are seen in patients with multiple sclerosis, Wilson disease, and cerebrovascular disease. ET is also confused with Parkinson's, so be sure to learn the difference between an action tremor and a resting tremor.

PPx: None

MoD: Unknown, and no genes have been identified in familial cases

Dx:
1. Clinical exam with symmetrical (usually) action tremor

Tx/Mgmt:
1. Propranolol (beta agonist activity)
2. Primidone (barbiturate)
3. Gabapentin, topiramate, mirtazapine for refractory cases

B. Acute Dystonia

Buzz Words: Abnormal posturing/position + worse with movement + neuroleptic exposure

99 AR
Basal Ganglia Video

Clinical Presentation: Acute dystonia does not refer to a single clinical entity, but is instead a product of a variety of underlying causes. Dystonias are involuntary muscle contractions resulting in abnormal postures and movements and can be limited to one part of the body, one side of the body, or most/all of the body (generalized). The list of underlying causes is large and includes neonatal hypoxia, kernicterus, AIDS, lysosomal storage disorders, and neurodegenerative diseases like Huntington's, PSP, and Parkinson's. The most commonly encountered dystonias are those restricted to parts of the body like the neck (torticollis), orbicularis oculi (blepharospasm), and hand (writer's cramp). Another important category is the dystonia caused by neuroleptics.

PPx: N/A

MoD: Variable due to multiple underlying pathologies. Neuroleptic induced dystonia is likely caused by antagonism of the D2 receptor. Haloperidol, fluphenazine, and metoclopramide are commonly associated with dystonias.

99 AR

Side Effects of Antipsychotics

Dx:

1. Clinical exam with repetitive, unnatural spasmodic movements (neuroleptic associated dystonia most commonly involves muscles around mouth, the tongue, or the neck)

Tx/Mgmt:

1. For neuroleptic associated dystonia, stop the offending agent and try diphenhydramine or benztropine

C. Tourette Syndrome

Buzz Words: Repetitive sniffing/snorting/vocalization + compulsive behavior + ADHD

Clinical Presentation: Tics are sudden, involuntary, stereotyped motor movements or vocalizations that are accompanied by an irresistible urge relieved by movement. Tourette's is the most severe tic syndrome and is characterized by multiple motor and vocal tics. The disorder begins in childhood, has a male predominance, and is associated with ADHD and obsessive-compulsive behavior. Like Sydenham chorea, a portion of Tourette cases are related to streptococcal infection (PANDAS—pediatric autoimmune neuropsychiatric disorders with streptococcal infection). Tics may arise from cryptococcal infection.

QUICK TIPS

Sydenham chorea = chorea of face/hands/feet after childhood infection with group A streptococcus

PPx: None

MoD: Unknown; may involve abnormalities of dopamine signaling in the caudate (levodopa makes symptoms worse; haloperidol makes symptoms better)

Dx:

1. Multiple motor and vocal tics
2. Tics occur many times/day
3. Onset before 21
4. Location, number, type, severity of tics change over time
5. Not explained by medication/substance/medical condition

In one-half of adolescents, the tics will subside before adulthood.

Tx/Mgmt:

1. Alpha2 adrenergic agonists (clonidine and guanfacine)
2. Antipsychotics (haloperidol, pimozide, risperidone)
3. Hyperactivity treated with methylphenidate or clonidine

Sleep Disorders

Sleep disorders are classified into insomnias (problems with falling asleep), hypersomnias (sleeping too much), or parasomnias (problems during sleep). The most commonly tested sleep disorder is narcolepsy (hypersomnia), which should be the number one take-home point for this chapter. For the other sleep disorders, get a sense of how one differentiates itself from the other, as the Buzz Words are relatively easy to pick. Mechanism of disease and diagnostic steps are less important.

In order to understand sleep disorders, one must learn the normal sleep-wake cycle. There are four stages of sleep:

- Stage 1 (non-rapid eye movement [REM]): Theta waves, muscle tone relaxed, eye movements—slow
- Stage 2 (non-REM): K complexes and sleep spindles with no eye movements and little muscle movement
- Stage 3 (non-REM): Delta sleep, low frequency, high voltage, slow wave sleep, deep sleep, most restful sleep, no dream recall
- Stage REM (R): Slow, fast voltage on the EEG, **no muscle tone** and REM, less restful than stage 3–4, saw tooth waves, vivid dream recall

A. Primary Insomnia (≥4 Weeks)

Buzz Words: Fatigue + memory impairment + worries about sleep + sleep interference despite **adequate opportunity to sleep**

Clinical Presentation: Patient is not able to sleep, and this has been going on for 4 weeks. Memory impairment here is caused by lack of sleep and not due to dementia. Also, there should be no other more likely diagnosis; primary insomnia is a diagnosis of exclusion.

PPx: Good sleep hygiene

MoD: Unknown

Dx:

1. Sleep diary
2. Psych evaluation (primary insomnia cannot be 2/2 another psych condition)

Tx/Mgmt:

1. Educate about sleep hygiene first, stimulus control therapy, relaxation, then CBT
2. Benzos (reduce sleep latency and increase slow wave sleep), such as temazepam
3. Nonbenzo hypnotics—Zolpidem, esZopiclone, and Zaleplon (three ZZZs for sleeping)
4. Antidepressants such as doxepin
5. Ramelteon (melatonin receptor agonist)

> **QUICK TIPS**
>
> Zolpidem, eszopiclone, and zaleplon are GABA_A receptor agonists.

B. Narcolepsy (>3 Months)

Buzz Words: Excessive daytime sleepiness + REM during naps + cataplexy (loss of muscle tone after laughter or extreme emotion) + hallucinations + sleep paralysis when waking up → narcolepsy

Clinical Presentation: Narcolepsy is the most commonly tested sleeping disorder on the shelf. It is also one of the most recognizable diseases, with patients sometimes presenting with cataplexy and sleep paralysis. Because it is so commonly tested, make sure you know the Buzz Words, mechanism and steps of treatment, and management very well.

PPx: N/A

MoD: Loss of hypocretin in hypothalamus

Dx:

1. Sleep diary
2. Sleep EEG

Tx/Mgmt:

1. Amphetamine (i.e., dextroamphetamine)
2. Modafinil/armodafinil

3. Sodium oxybate or desipramine (treatment of cataplexy)
4. Amphetamine-like medicines—methylphenidate
5. SSRIs and tricyclic antidepressants (TCAs)

C. Idiopathic Hypersomnia

Buzz Words: Excessive daytime sleepiness + prolonged nocturnal sleep episodes + frequent urges to nap

Clinical Presentation: Idiopathic hypersomnia is rarely tested, but you may see this as a distractor answer choice.

PPx: None

MoD: Idiopathic

Dx:

1. Sleep diary
2. Sleep EEG

Tx/Mgmt:

1. Improve sleep hygiene
2. Stimulant meds

D. Kleine Levin Syndrome

Buzz Words: Hypersomnia + hyperphagia + hypersexuality + aggression → Klein Levin syndrome

Clinical Presentation: Klein Levin syndrome is characterized by the three H's: hypersomnia, hyperphagia, and hypersexuality. This is a rare disease, so only the Buzz Words are likely to be tested.

PPx: None

MoD: Unknown

Dx:

1. Clinical exam
2. CT/MRI to r/o structural lesions

Tx/Mgmt:

1. Stimulants (e.g., modafinil)

E. Circadian Rhythm Sleep Disorders

For these disorders, PPx and Dx are not tested. Instead, know the Buzz Words, mechanism, and treatment for each circadian rhythm sleep disorder subtype.

MoD: Dysregulation of suprachiasmatic nucleus in the hypothalamus

Buzz Words for subtypes:

1. **Delayed sleep phase disorder (night owl)**
   a. Delay in sleep onset and awakening times with preserved quality and duration caused by puberty, caffeine, irregular schedules
   b. Treat with **light therapy, melatonin,** and chronotherapy

2. **Advanced sleep phase disorder (early sleeper)**
   a. Normal duration and quality with earlier onset and awakening associated with older age
   b. Treat with evening phototherapy
3. **Shift-work disorder**
   a. Misalignment of circadian rhythm from work
   b. Tx with bright light therapy to adapt to night shift and modafinil to stay awake
4. **Jet lag**
   a. Sleep disturbance from traveling
   b. Self-limiting

F. Sleepwalking (Somnambulism)

Buzz Words: Simple to complex behaviors during slow-wave sleep (deep sleep) + eyes open and glassy look + confusion on awakening with amnesia of event → sleep walking

Clinical Presentation: Rarely tested but often seen as a distractor answer choice

PPx: None

MoD: Unknown

Dx:
1. History from coinhabitant

Tx/Mgmt:
1. Clonazepam (Benzos)
2. TCA

G. Sleep Terrors (Stage 3)

Buzz Words: Episodes of sudden arousal in complete terror with screaming during **slow-wave sleep** + return to sleep w/o awakening + **no memory** of episode

No memory because it occurs in stage 3 of sleep, where no memory of dreams occur

Clinical Presentation: Very frequently tested because it is very similar to nightmare disorder. The key difference is that patients with sleep terrors do not remember their dream, whereas those with nightmare disorder do.

PPx: None

MoD: Related to sympathetic hyperactivation and increased muscle tone

Dx:
1. Clinical exam
2. Sleep diary

Tx/Mgmt:
1. Benzos
2. Protect from injuring themselves during episodes

H. Nightmare Disorder

Buzz Words: Frightening dreams that cause awakening with vivid recall + related to posttraumatic stress disorder (PTSD) and in women

Clinical Presentation: Patients with nightmare disorder remember their nightmare (as opposed to patients with sleep terrors).

PPx: Tx of PTSD

MoD: Related to prior trauma

Dx:
1. Clinical exam
2. Sleep diary

Tx/Mgmt:
1. Imagery rehearsal therapy
2. Antidepressants for severe cases

Not treated with benzos, because this occurs in different stage of sleep

I. REM Behavior Disorder

Buzz Words: Muscle atonia during REM sleep and complex motor activity with dream mentation + sleep talking, yelling, kicking spouse (aka periodic leg movement disorder) + recall of dreams

Clinical Presentation: A very commonly tested disease. The story will always be told by patient's significant other, who gives the most important Buzz Word of kicking/punching during sleep.

PPx: None

MoD: Can be associated with Parkinson's or be idiopathic

Dx:
1. Clinical exam
2. Sleep diary

Tx/Mgmt:
1. R/o medical conditions (Fe anemia, chronic kidney disease, neuropathy)
2. Clonazepam (first line of treatment)
3. Dopamine agonists (i.e., pramipexole, ropinirole)
4. Carbamazepine
5. Levodopa

J. Restless Legs Syndrome

Buzz Words: Irresistible urge to move legs + urge is relieved when patient moves legs + impairs sleep + leads to nocturnal awakenings

Versus periodic limb movements in sleep (PLMS) or periodic limb movement disorder (PLMD), where patient has repetitive 30 seconds twitching of legs or arms during sleep, and is associated with REM behavior disorder

Clinical Presentation: Restless legs syndrome (RLS) is considered a movement disorder instead of a sleep disorder. However, it can cause one to present like a sleep disorder (e.g., nonrestful sleep) due to an irresistible urge to move the legs. Thus it is important to have RLS in your differential for sleep disorders.

PPx: None

MoD: Unknown but may be related to dopamine dysfunction

Dx:
1. History from patient and coinhabitant
2. Polysomnography to r/o PLMD

Tx/Mgmt:
1. Pramipexole, ropinirole
2. Rotigotine patch
3. Gabapentin
4. Iron supplements if Fe anemia

Seizures

Seizure is an important topic in neurology and rarely, if ever, evaluated by psychiatrists. However, these may appear on your psychiatry for two reasons: (1) many of the mood stabilizer drugs (e.g., valproate, carbamazepine) are antiepileptic drugs (AEDs), and (2) some patients fake seizure symptoms for primary or secondary gain, and may be referred to a psychiatrist. For the purposes of the psychiatry shelf, focus on Buzz Words and types of AEDs used.

With respect to organizing principles of seizures, know the following: First, recognize that ALL seizures are caused by synchronized neuronal discharge. Second, recognize that many seizures start in the temporal lobe. Some may go on to stay in one area of the brain and are thus called **partial** seizures. Some may go on to recruit neurons of the whole brain, and are therefore called **generalized** seizures. Oftentimes, the only way to diagnose the epilepsy syndromes is by EEG recording, but there are certain clinical clues you can use to help you.

This subsection is low-yield for psychiatry shelf so feel free to skip if pressed for time. Otherwise, spend no more than 45 minutes perusing the material.

Partial Seizures

A. Simple Partial Seizure (Focal Seizure)

Buzz Words: Preserved consciousness + tonic/clonic movements of an isolated part of the body + 10–20 seconds + no postictal period

Clinical Presentation: In simple partial seizures, the consciousness is preserved. Tonic or clonic movements involving most of the face, neck, and extremities and lasting 10–20 seconds can be seen. There is also no postictal period.

PPx: None

MoD: Synchronized neuronal discharge

Dx:

1. Localized spike and sharp waves on EEG

Tx/Mgmt:

1. First line: Carbamazepine and valproic acid
2. Lamotrigine

B. Complex Partial Seizure (Focal Seizure With Consciousness Disturbance)

Buzz Words: Impaired consciousness + tonic/clonic movements of an isolated part of the body + 10–20 seconds + no postictal period

Clinical Presentation: Similar presentation to simple partial seizures but have impaired consciousness

PPx: None

MoD: Synchronized neuronal discharge

Dx:

1. EEG → Anterior temporal lobe shows sharp waves or focal spikes

Tx/Mgmt:

1. First line: valproic acid, carbamazepine
2. Lamotrigine

Generalized Seizures

Generalized seizures usually distort activity in the whole or large part of the brain, which is usually characteristic on EEG recording. By definition, generalized seizures impair consciousness, so patients have **no memory** of the event. Most begin in childhood, and for many patients will go away by adulthood. For those in which it does not go away, they will require lifelong treatment with medications such as valproic acid, lamotrigine, and topiramate. Although there are many new AEDs that are considered first line treatment, the shelf exam questions will likely only expect you to know the three mentioned here.

A. Absence Seizure (Petite Mal)

Buzz Words: Blank stare + pause in activities for a few seconds + induced by hyperventilation + no memory of event

Clinical Presentation: Absence seizures are more common in girls, rare in children less than 5 years, and rarely last longer than 30 seconds. There is no aura or postictal state. They commonly present with a blank stare that appears benign (e.g., no other body movements).

This is the commonly tested seizure, and the treatment modality (ethosuximide) is frequently asked on the shelf.

PPx: None

MoD: Dysfunction of T-type calcium channels

Dx:
1. 3 per second (3 Hz) typical spike and wave discharges

Tx/Mgmt:
1. Ethosuximide
2. Valproic acid

B. Juvenile Myoclonic Epilepsy (JME)

Buzz Words: Quick, myoclonic jerks of arms + teenager + occurs in morning + followed by clonic-tonic generalized seizure

Clinical Presentation: Classic presentation is a teenager who seizes in the morning

PPx: None

MoD: Synchronized neuronal discharge

Dx:
1. EEG

Tx/Mgmt: Valproic acid

C. Idiopathic Generalized Epilepsy

Buzz Words: Loss of consciousness + skeletal muscles tense, alternating stiffening and movement + whole body movement

Clinical Presentation: Presents as frequent Tonic-Clonic seizures (aka grand mal). The patient's muscles will start to contract and relax rapidly, causing convulsions.

PPx: None

MoD: Synchronized neuronal discharge

Dx:
1. EEG

Tx/Mgmt:
1. Phenytoin
2. Valproic acid

GUNNER PRACTICE

1. An 82-year-old woman is brought to the physician by her husband because of an 8-month history of confusion and "seeing things." Most recently, her husband heard her converse with "pleasant little fairies" sitting in the living room, although there was nobody in the living room at that time. Her activities of daily living have gradually become more difficult to perform independently. She

currently takes lisinopril for hypertension and a multivitamin. She had her appendix taken out when she was 22. Her last job was as manager of a local restaurant. Her vitals show a BP of 130/90, pulse is 90/min, temperature is 98.9°F. Heart is regular rate and rhythm and lungs are clear to auscultation. Upon ambulation, patient gait is narrow and slow. She appears to have a reactive affect, but she is unable to draw the hands of a clock accurately. Complete metabolic panel was within normal limits. What is the most likely diagnosis?

A. Schizophrenia
B. Schizophreniform
C. Schizoaffective
D. Lewy body dementia
E. Vascular dementia

2. A 43-year-old woman comes to her primary care doctor complaining of an 8-month history of fatigue and trouble sleeping. Every night, after she goes to bed, there is an uncomfortable feeling in both her legs that can keep her up for several hours. When she wakes up, she complains that she has had "too little sleep" and is concerned that her performance at work is being adversely affected. She is worried about doing better to get a desired promotion. Her sleep is interrupted until she awakens from her alarm, although her boyfriend has complained about occasional loud snores. The only medication she currently takes is a multivitamin. She had surgery 10 years ago to fix a right ankle fracture. Her vital signs are within normal limits, and her BMI is 29 kg/m². On examination, there is a well-healed incisional scar that runs vertically on the right ankle. Quadriceps, tibialis anterior, extensor hallucis longus, gastrocnemius/soleus muscles are 5/5 strength bilaterally. Superficial peroneal, deep peroneal, sural, saphenous, and posterior tibial nerve distributions are intact to light touch on both legs. She states that she is "a little anxious" about her condition, and her affect is congruent to stated mood. Sometimes she gets exasperated about not being able to fall asleep right away and tries to "walk it off." Complete blood count is within the reference range. What is the most likely diagnosis?

A. Generalized anxiety disorder
B. Normal response to stress
C. Obstructive sleep apnea
D. Restless legs syndrome
E. Sequelae of surgery

3. A 77-year-old woman is brought to the neurologist by her son because of memory loss for the past 4 weeks. Just last week, she forgot to turn off the faucet in her kitchen sink before leaving the house to run errands. When the son calls to check in on her, she sometimes calls him by her husband's name. Her husband died 11 months ago, and she reports being constantly distraught by the thought of him over this time period. At baseline, she continues to live alone, do her own chores, and drive to the nearest grocery store, and was doing well until recently. Her vital signs are within normal limits. She walks with a cane to alleviate knee pain and reports her mood as "I'm feeling down." Her affect is congruent with her stated mood, but she denies suicidal ideation. She still enjoys knitting and reading, but does not do these activities as frequently. What is the most appropriate next step in management?

A. Refer to a psychiatrist

B. Start a selective serotonin reuptake inhibitor

C. Recommend cognitive behavior therapy

D. Mini-mental state examination

E. Head CT

ANSWERS: What Would Gunner Jess/Jim Do?

1. WWGJD? An 82-year-old woman is brought to the physician by her husband because of an 8-month history of confusion and "seeing things." Most recently, her husband heard her converse with "pleasant little fairies" sitting in the living room, although there was nobody in the living room at that time. Her activities of daily living have gradually become more difficult to perform independently. She currently takes lisinopril for hypertension and a multivitamin. She had her appendix taken out when she was 22. Her last job was as manager of a local restaurant. Her vitals show a BP of 130/90, pulse is 90/min, temperature is 98.9F. Heart is regular rate and rhythm and lungs are clear to auscultation. Upon ambulation, patient gait is narrow and slow. She appears to have a reactive affect, but she is unable to draw the hands of a clock accurately. Complete metabolic panel was within normal limits. What is the most likely diagnosis?

Answer: D. Lewy body dementia

Explanation: Lewy body dementia is a combination of parkinsonian signs/symptoms, lilliputian hallucinations, and dementia. There are two important considerations when answering this question. First, are the woman's symptoms psych or neuro related? The clue of her being "unable to draw the hands of a clock accurately" suggests dementia. Also, her "reactive affect," defined as affect that changes appropriately to situation or mood, makes schizophrenia and its range of similar disorders less likely. Patients with schizophrenia, for instance, would typically be described as having a "blunt" or "flat" affect, one of the disorder's defining negative symptoms 2/2 too little dopamine in the mesocortical pathway. Thus A–C can be ruled out. Second, it is important to recognize the Buzz Word "pleasant little..." visual hallucinations. Visual hallucinations described as pleasant and "little" or "small" on the shelf exam are lilliputian hallucinations, until proven otherwise, and are pathognomonic for Lewy body dementia.

A. Schizophrenia → Incorrect. Although patient clearly has been experiencing visual hallucinations for ≥6 months, there are other clues in the question stem, such as her "reactive affect" or "narrow and slow" gait that suggests different pathology. Schizophrenic patients will classically exhibit negative

gg AR

Example of Lewy Body Dementia: Robin Williams

symptoms, such as a flat or blunted affect, in the question stem.

B. Schizophreniform → Incorrect. Schizophreniform disorder is diagnosed when patients have the signs and symptoms of schizophrenia from 1 to 6 months. This answer choice should immediately be eliminated since symptoms have been ongoing for 8 months.

C. Schizoaffective → Incorrect. Schizoaffective disorder is defined as mood swings (either mania or depression) in the setting of psychotic episodes. Since patient does not exhibit any mood swings, this answer can be ruled out.

E. Vascular dementia → Incorrect. Although the patient had signs of dementia (e.g., unable to draw the hands of a clock), she had other signs, such as "narrow and slow" gait that point to Lewy body dementia. Question stems in which vascular dementia is the correct answer will explicitly highlight how the patient has had a stepwise decline (e.g., gets worse with every infarct). There was no stepwise decline reported in this question stem.

2. WWGJD? A 43-year-old woman comes to her primary care doctor complaining of an 8-month history of fatigue and trouble sleeping. Every night, after she goes to bed, there is an uncomfortable feeling in both her legs that can keep her up for several hours. When she wakes up, she complains that she has had "too little sleep" and is concerned that her performance at work is being adversely affected. She is worried about doing better to get a desired promotion. Her sleep is interrupted until she awakens from her alarm, although her boyfriend has complained about occasional loud snores. The only medication she currently takes is a multivitamin. She had surgery ten years ago to fix a right ankle fracture. Her vital signs are within normal limits, and her BMI is 29 kg/m². On examination, there is a well-healed incisional scar that runs vertically on the right ankle. Quadriceps, tibialis anterior, extensor hallucis longus, gastrocnemius/soleus muscles are 5/5 strength bilaterally. Superficial peroneal, deep peroneal, sural, saphenous, and posterior tibial nerve distributions are intact to light touch on both legs. She states that she is "a little anxious" about her condition, and her affect is congruent to stated mood. Sometimes, she gets exasperated about not being able to fall asleep right away and tries to "walk it off." Complete blood count is within the reference range. What is the most likely diagnosis?

Answer: D. Restless legs syndrome

Explanation: This patient has restless legs syndrome, most clearly highlighted by the "uncomfortable feeling" in her legs that she tries to "walk" off in order to fall asleep. Restless legs syndrome is pretty straightforward to diagnose. However, questions on the shelf attempt to tire out or confuse the examinee by adding a lot of extraneous information, such as her history of ankle fracture, physical exam findings, and her "occasional loud snore." It is imperative to recognize important Buzz Words and move on without spending too much time reading the question stem. Remember you only have 90 seconds per question (150 minutes for a 100-question test), and your first instinct is usually correct.

A. Generalized anxiety disorder → Incorrect. GAD is perhaps the trickiest out of the incorrect answer choices. The criteria for diagnosing GAD is at least three WATCHERS symptoms (**W**orry that is excessive, **A**nxiety, **T**ense muscles, **C**oncentration decreased, **H**yperarousal/irritability, **E**nergy decreased, **R**estlessness, **S**leep disturbance and somatic manifestation) for ≥6 months. In this question stem, the patient reports decreased energy, restlessness, and sleep disturbance, which may appear as meeting diagnostic criteria. However, GAD cannot be diagnosed if there is another more likely diagnosis. In this case, the patient's restlessness is 2/2 to a "feeling" that she can walk off; this suggests restless legs syndrome. In addition, her sleep disturbance is a consequence of this feeling in her legs and not her anxiety. In addition, the patient does not exhibit excessive worry and cannot be said to be anxious. She is distraught by not being able to fall asleep, and she is worried about her job performance, but this is a normal reaction to her condition. Folks with GAD will frequently present in the question stem, worrying about multiple things in their professional and personal life when the degree of worrying is not justified.

B. Normal response to stress → Incorrect. Although the patient's anxiety is a normal response to her restless legs syndrome, the feeling in her legs is not normal.

C. Obstructive sleep apnea → Incorrect. Patient only occasionally snores and is not yet obese with a BMI of 29 kg/m². In addition, OSA would not explain the restlessness in her legs.

   E. Sequelae of surgery → Incorrect. Although there was a lot in the question stem written about the surgery and physical exam findings, the procedure was on the right leg whereas the symptoms are bilateral. Surgical procedures of the lower extremity can sometimes lead to intractable pain (e.g., complex regional pain syndrome), but what the patient is describing in the question stem is not painful.

3. WWGJD? A 77-year-old woman is brought to the neurologist by her son because of memory loss for the past four weeks. Just last week, she forgot to turn off the faucet in her kitchen sink before leaving the house to run errands. When the son calls to check in on her, she sometimes calls him by her husband's name. Her husband died 11 months ago and she reports being constantly distraught by the thought of him over this time period. At baseline, she continues to live alone, do her own chores, and drive to the nearest grocery store, and was doing well until recently. His vital signs are within normal limits. She walks with a cane to alleviate knee pain and reports her mood as "I'm feeling down." Her affect is congruent with her stated mood but she denies suicidal ideation. She still enjoys knitting and reading, but does not do these activities as frequently. What is the most appropriate next step in management?

Answer: D. Mini-mental state examination

   Explanation: The neurology questions on the psych shelf try to trick you by tempting you with psychiatric diagnostic steps and treatment options when the underlying pathology is neurologic. In this case, the patient has pseudodementia (depression symptoms early in the course of degenerative dementia) and needs to be worked up for dementia. The first step is to do an MMSE. There is not enough information available yet to recommend therapy.

   A. Refer to a psychiatrist → Incorrect. The patient's symptoms still appear to be more neurologic than psychiatric. Referral to a psychiatrist would be appropriate if patient's chief complaint was sadness and reported anhedonia. If patient reported active suicidal ideation, it would be appropriate to consider referral to the ED so that patient can be hospitalized.

B. Start a selective serotonin reuptake inhibitor →
   Incorrect. Not enough information has been discovered to recommend therapy. Patient also does not
   yet meet the criteria for major depression disorder,
   which requires patient to report anhedonia. This
   answer choice should immediately be ruled out.
C. Recommend cognitive behavior therapy → Incorrect.
   Again, not enough information has been discovered
   to recommend therapy. Patient also does not yet
   meet the criteria for major depression disorder,
   which requires patient to report anhedonia. This
   answer choice should immediately be ruled out.
E. Head CT → Incorrect. Head imaging with CT or
   MRI may be necessary as subsequent diagnostic
   steps to rule out cerebrovascular disease. However,
   patient needs to be evaluated by the MMSE first
   before physician can proceed with ordering tests.

Gunner Jim's Guide to Exam Day Success

Hao-Hua Wu and Leo Wang

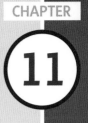

11

Do these three things to perform well on any shelf:
1. Master one review book.
2. Do as many quality questions as you can.
3. Excel like a Gunner.

"Master one review book."

Psychiatry clerkship rotations range from 2 to 6 weeks. That is not enough time to peruse multiple review books. The most important thing you can do prior to the start of your rotation is to identify the resource that best covers the material of the psychiatry shelf. Once you have picked something, stick with it. The point of using a review book is to get familiarized with the scope of the exam.

Most of your learning occurs when you complete questions, so don't be discouraged if you cannot memorize every word of your review book like you did for Step 1. Instead, use your review book as a point of reference and annotate the margins.

If you see one topic come up on multiple chapters (or maybe even multiple shelf exams), make sure to write down the page numbers where it appears and flip to those pages every time you review. The more connections you make, the more you will master.

In addition, highlight themes that keep coming up. Any time patients in the question stem have recently changed their medication regimen, suspect the medication change as the cause of their symptoms until proven otherwise. These organizing principles transcend individual topics and can help you do well on any shelf exam test question.

"Do as many quality questions as you can."

The key to success is practicing in an environment that simulates the pressure of test day. And nothing simulates that pressure better than taking practice questions under stringent time constraints.

After you identify your review book, select as many authoritative question banks as you can. We recommend Gunner Practice, UWorld, and NBME Clinical Science practice exams. Do at least 10 questions a day under timed conditions (1.5 minutes a question), starting on the first day of your rotation.

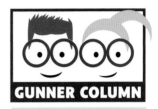

GUNNER COLUMN

Remember, you can complete the same question multiple times in the course of study! In fact, it is recommended that you retry the questions you got wrong in the first place, just so that you know you will get it right on the test.

It is also important that the questions you complete are of high quality. This means that the length and content of the question stems reflect what you would actually see on test day. Many question bank resources are too easy (giving you a false sense of confidence) or ask about material that would not show up on the exam (wasting your time).

Once you have selected your question bank resources, count the total number of questions and divide it by the number of days you have available to study. Then make sure you set a study plan where you can make at least two passes through your questions. The first pass is completion of all available questions. The second pass is completion of all the questions you got wrong or made a lucky guess on during your first pass. Seeing how many of the second pass questions you get correct should be a nice confidence boost leading into exam day.

As you do questions, jot down patterns associated with the chief complaint. NBME question writers are instructed to write questions with a chief complaint that can plausibly be associated with at least five different diseases. Sharpen your differential after you read a question's first sentence, and then use Buzz Words to narrow down your diagnosis. Once you reach your diagnosis, you will either be done with the question or have to draw upon knowledge of Prophylaxis (PPx), Mechanism of Disease (MoD), Diagnostic Steps (Dx), and Treatment/Management (Tx/Mgmt). "Excel like a Gunner."

How you take notes for the questions you complete is imperative to success.

The most effective strategy is to pick **one** take-home point for every question you complete and record it on an Excel sheet specific for your clinical rotation.

For instance, if you answer a question incorrectly about the treatment of schizophrenia causing metabolic syndrome, write "Tx of schizophrenia—metabolic syndrome" in column A of your Excel sheet and then "Olanzapine" in column B of your Excel sheet. This allows you to create an immediate, pseudo-flashcard. When you review this material the following week, you can put your cursor over column A, say the answer out loud, and check your answer by shifting your cursor to column B. This saves time and emphasizes the most important takeaway for each question. You can also make your own flash cards on the Gunner Goggles iOS app.

If you understand everything in the question and answer choices, don't record it in the Excel sheet.

If you don't understand multiple things in the question and answer choices, record the most important takeaway point and move on. For test day, it is better to be confident in what you know well than to undermine your confidence by fixating on what you are weak at.

By test day, you should have one Excel sheet that contains one important take-home point from every question you were unsure about. The tabs on the bottom should be organized by question bank resource. This Excel would ideally only take 3–4 hours to review, and is something you would go over the day before the exam.

Last but not least, **trust the process.** Students often enter test day anxious and overwhelmed, which can cause them to second guess their answer choices. Trust the process—trust that you will have covered everything in leading up to the shelf exam and have some faith in your answer selections; for these reasons, don't second guess yourself. Your first instinct is usually right.

In summary: Read. Apply. Review. And prepare for success on test day!

Index

Note: Page numbers followed by *f,* indicate figures; *t,* tables, *b,* boxes.